MW00986430

Survivalist Family
Prepared Americans for a Strong America

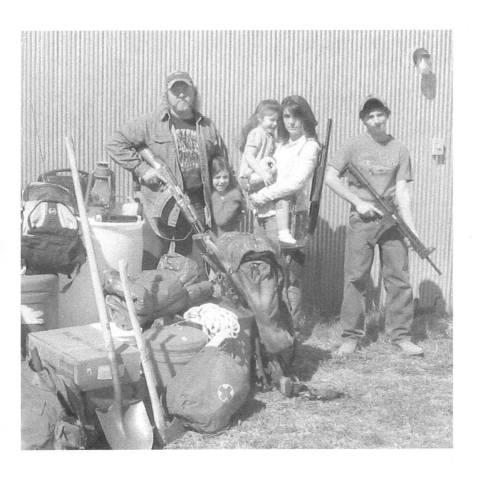

Survivalist Family
Prepared Americans for a Strong America
Author: Joe Fox
www.vikingpreparedness.com

Copyright ©Joe Fox 2010
All rights reserved

ISBN: 978-1-935018-25-4

Without limiting the rights under copyright reserved above, no part of this publication may be reproduced, stored in or introduced into a retrieval system, or transmitted, in any form, or by any means (electronic, mechanical, photocopying, recording, or otherwise), without the prior written permission of both the copyright owner and the above publisher of this book.

Published by:
Five Stones Publishing,
a division of:
The International Localization Network
ILNcenter.com

The publisher does not have any control over and does not assume any responsibility for author or third-party Web sites or their content.

"No matter how much the federal government, the state, or local officials do to prepare, we can't do it alone – individuals and families must do their part to be ready in case of an emergency." - W. Craig Fugate Administrator of the Federal Emergency Management Agency

Go to the ant, you sluggard! Consider her ways and be wise.
Which, having no guide, overseer or ruler, provides her supplies in the summer and gathers her food in the harvest.

How long will you sleep, O sluggard?
When will you arise out of your sleep?

Yet a little sleep, a little slumber, a little folding of the hands to sleep: So shall your need come upon you as a highwayman and your want as an armed man.
                    - Proverbs 6:6 - 11

For Morri

Table of Contents

Foreword

I don't often find myself agreeing with other preparedness writers. All too often, so many of the preparedness books written in the last decade have been what I call a "book of lists." Usually these are just lists of things to purchase. New people come into the movement and too frequently the question is asked, "What do I need to buy?" While I'm in no way disputing the need to stockpile items, the typical American mindset of "buying" your way out of a problem doesn't always work well in a survival situation. A fine balance between stockpiling items and learning skill sets must be obtained. More times than not, new survivalists never take their preparations any further than "buying things." This ought not to be so!

I do find myself agreeing with Joe on a regular basis, both on his internet posts and in reading this book. Having met Joe I can tell you that he is a DOER. In this book when he says "your child must be physically fit" know that his children ARE physically fit. When he says "you must be able to talk with your wife..." know that his wife IS fully with him in their family preparedness endeavors. I can certainly appreciate people who practice what they preach.

Joe has written an excellent book here, perfect for the beginner, but with just enough nuggets of knowledge to also satisfy those of us that have been around the block for a decade or three. You will enjoy this book and more importantly it should help you greatly in your preparedness journey.

Robert Henry
www.survivalreport.net

Introduction

We live in unsettled times. We cannot turn on the television or the radio without hearing about some disaster or incident which has negatively altered the lives of so many people. Our government attempts to inform and educate us while simultaneously warning us of some future threat and telling us "everything will be okay." The mixed messages we receive, the sad news we see and hear, all combine at times to create a sense of dread mixed with hopelessness.

Things should not be so! We should all live happy and hopeful lives. We should all finish our days knowing that everything in our personal world will be okay. We should all be able to sleep soundly at night knowing that we have done everything we can to ensure that we and our loved ones will be able to deal with whatever Life throws at us. And let's face it – sometimes we do get some interesting curve balls thrown our way.

The book you now hold in your hands will help you to prepare for those curve balls. This is not some gloom and doom "The World Is Ending!" book. This is more of a manual that will help you to take action – to take positive steps that will allow you to ensure your loved ones and indeed, your neighbors, come through any crises that may occur.

As you will read, I have been at this for a long time. I have read almost every other book in the genre – some are very good, but most left me very frustrated. I think you will enjoy this treatment of the subject of family preparedness. I think you will learn new things – useful things. That you do so is my hope; that you take steps to ensure your own preparedness and the preparedness of those around you is my prayer.

Prepared Americans for a Strong America!

Joe Fox
March 2010
www.vikingpreparedness.com

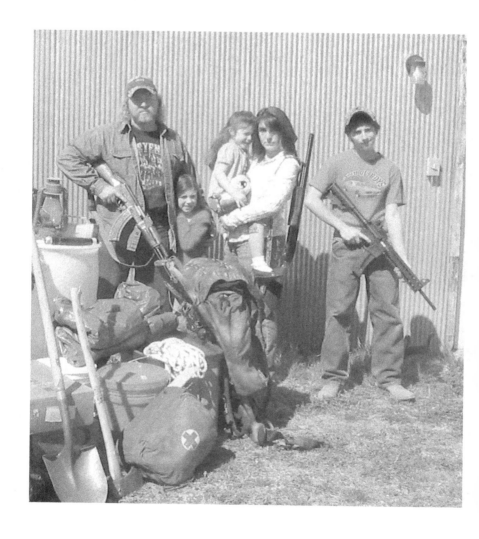

BEGINNINGS

Just what IS a "survivalist family"?

I suppose some people shudder at the very thought! Watch enough television and you'll see that the media's version of a survivalist family is a dirty, ignorant clan living in a remote ramshackle log cabin. It will consist of a fat, bearded, camouflage-wearing, tobacco chewing, over domineering misogynist running roughshod over his cowering mouse of a wife who is trying to raise filthy little barefoot ragamuffins who run around spouting racist right-wing propaganda they picked up from "Pa".

Well, who would want to read about THAT? Certainly not you. Instead of "survivalist family" we could say "prepared family" or talk about "family preparedness" but that is just so politically correct it makes me gag. Just because the media don't like survivalists and therefore vilify them does not mean we have to change our language. For our purposes, the Survivalist Family is defined as, "A multi-generational group of people living in one house (usually consisting of a father, mother and their offspring) who take positive steps as a cohesive group to prepare for possible future negative situations and circumstances beyond their control."

We say "multi-generational" because if it's a man and a woman they are really a couple – not a family in the truest sense of the word. It's actually easier for a couple to prepare than a family. Just because a family in our definition usually consists of a father, mother and children does not mean that a single mom with two boys is not a family – they are. I said "usually". So do not get hung up on people – focus on what they do. They take *positive* steps to prepare *as a group* for future bad times.

Where do Survivalist Families live? Everywhere - in city apartments, in suburban split-levels, in country farm houses and yes, even in remote log cabins surrounded by deep, dark woods.

What kinds of jobs do Mom and Dad have? Every kind imaginable - Dad could be senior geologist for the Department of Agriculture, a grocer, a mechanic, or a computer programmer. Mom could be a nuclear scientist, a secretary or a stay-at-home-mom.

In a nutshell - they are average, every-day American families who have taken the decision to prepare for emergencies. The level to which they prepare varies greatly and is not always obvious. You probably have some Survivalist Families in your neighborhood and do not even realize it.

Most are not very forthcoming about their preparations. One reason is fear of being labeled a "survivalist" and having friends and neighbors think them kooky. Some fear that when bad times come, their family could be at risk if others knew of their preparations. Someone who failed to prepare may try to take what they have or the government may requisition their supplies or any of a myriad of other reasons.

Why Prepare?

I suspect that the very fact you are reading this book indicates you have at least *some* interest in preparing. First of all - IT JUST MAKES SENSE. Our national infrastructure is relatively fragile - power goes out, water gets polluted, people get snowed in. My family lived in a town that was hit by a severe ice storm in 1996. Power lines went down all over the region. Not long after, our town's water pumps stopped working. Some people were without water and electricity in their homes for over a week. Think about that - no showers, no cooking, no washing clothes, no flushing toilets.

Every year towns all over this land are struck with hurricanes, tornados, floods, fires or other acts of God that place citizens into emergency situations. Basic services are disrupted, families are displaced, and life quickly becomes "different". Basic necessities suddenly become extremely valuable. Simple skills our grandparents had take on renewed importance.

Our economy is troubled. What if you lost your job tomorrow - how long could your family survive without a paycheck coming in? When would you run out of food, heat, etc? Being prepared with an adequate amount of food and basic supplies would allow you to stave of panic and take the time to focus on getting another good job.

We now all know there is a real terrorist threat to our nation. How will they strike again when they do? Will it affect you and your family? Perhaps. If the major highways were shut down for just a week or so the impact on communities would be enormous. Picture your local grocery store on the eve of an approaching winter storm. People mob the check out counters and soon there is no milk, bread, or batteries to be had. For a simple snowstorm. Imagine if the interstates were closed. Far fetched? Your government doesn't think so. Take some time to review the Red Cross, FEMA, and Department of Homeland Security websites.

Weapons of mass destruction are proliferating. Nuclear nations include: USA, Russia, China, England, France, India, Pakistan, North Korea, Israel and probably South Africa. Those are the ones we know about. Iran is trying hard to acquire nuclear material to construct weapons. Supposedly, accountability of Russian "suitcase nukes" has been lost. Terrorists have studied building radiological dispersion devices - the so-called "dirty bombs". Full-blown nuclear war is not out of the question. Even if it was conducted in other countries - it is possible that clouds of nuclear fallout would spread around the globe to your home town.

Want to consider more dire threats? Read your history. We live in the greatest nation on Earth - no doubt about it. But great nations do not last forever. They also do not usually change without a lot of turmoil - turmoil that would affect you and yours. We could be nuked, we could be invaded, or there could be another civil war. Life as you know could change - possibly for the worse.

If any of the above situations happen, will you and your family be prepared to deal with it or will you curl up into a fetal position, suck your thumb and cry for help? What if no one hears you or comes to your aid? During long term, major crises, there will not be a lot of help. The "helpers" will be overwhelmed trying to take care of themselves. It's up to you to prepare for yourself and your family. It is *your* responsibility.

My Journey

Why am I writing this book? What do I bring to the discussion? First and foremost, my family and I are survivalists. We have developed a systematic approach that has worked for us and I'd like to share it with you. I strongly believe in our nation and one of my mottos is, "Prepared Americans for a strong America". Simply put - I want you and your family to prepare for possible emergencies.

I have been "into preparedness" for my entire life. My father worked for a government agency that moved our family around to various overseas postings - always to underdeveloped nations. As such, we always had basic survival supplies in our homes - we never knew when things would just stop working. Things like electricity, water, transportation and so on. Our family was evacuated twice - once because of war and once because of floods. We had bug out bags and 72-hour kits before the terms were invented.

I was heavily involved in Boy Scouts and developed a love for the outdoors through many campouts, canoe trips, hikes, and so on. I picked up a lot of useful skills along the way. I was the first in my troop to earn the wilderness survival merit badge when it came out. I read every military survival manual in existence. For a variety of reasons, I became extremely interested in outdoor activities in general and wilderness survival in particular.

Entering college in the early 80's I became interested in "survivalism" and started gathering supplies, making plans and so forth. This time period was one of the high water marks for the survivalist movement and I was coming of age at that critical juncture.

Entering the Army upon graduation I matriculated from the light Infantry to Special Forces where I spent most of my career. I had the privilege of attending some of the best survival training available - all funded by the U.S. taxpayer and became, amongst other things, a certified SERE instructor (Survival, Evasion, Resistance, and Escape).

In the late 1990s I worked for a national intelligence agency and had insight into our government's real thoughts and preparations for Y2K. About all I will say about that is, "your government was very worried and took great measures to protect itself." I saw what was going on and really ramped up my family's preparation efforts. Thank God it was much ado about nothing - although some think the government merely used it as a practice run for possible contingencies down the road. Does the government know something you do not? Usually.

Around this time, my wife and I started hanging out on Internet survivalist and Y2K preparation boards and attending survivalist get-togethers with others we met mostly on the net. We met some colorful characters and had some interesting times with others of like mind. There *were* some weirdoes and paranoids at these gatherings but the vast majority of folks were just normal everyday people who wanted to make sure they came out on the other side of whatever life threw at them.

My wife had a similar upbringing to my own and spent large portions of her childhood growing up overseas. We met in college and took a backpacking course together. From that point forward, we "grew" together in the survivalist lifestyle although I did have to do some poking, prodding, cajoling and leading along the way.

We have three children whose upbringing allowed us to form many of the ideas and techniques in this book. Our children are all good students and active in sports, church activities and scouts. My wife and I are both scout leaders and have been so since our son was old enough to join Cub Scouts.

So, now you know where I'm coming from, a little about my and my family's background and why I'm writing this book. Let's now start into the nitty-gritty.

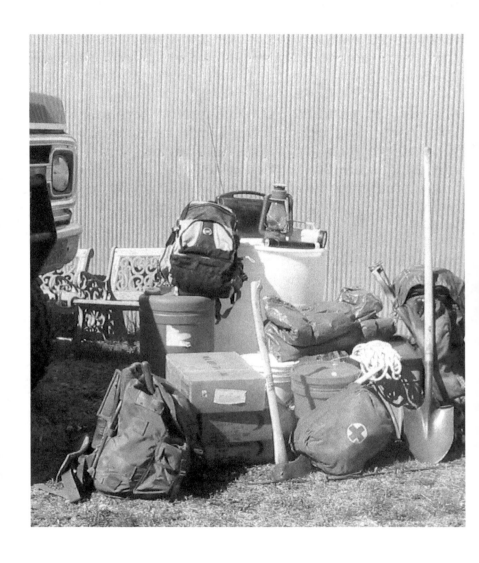

GETTING STARTED

The Basics

Later in this book we will cover Threat-based Planning where you will determine just what it is you need to prepare for. But for now, there are certain things every family should be able to do and areas you should definitely cover in your survival planning.

You must be able to take care of the basics. You should have a supply of food, water, and medicine adequate for your needs. You should have some basic equipment and an information packet. In any emergency basic services are the first things to be curtailed. It does not take a comet striking the earth for the grocery stores to run out of food or the water taps to quit working. Government entities are now recommending around three weeks of food, water and medicine - a three day supply in a 72-hour kit, a two weeks emergency supply in the home and a three day supply in your vehicle.

Water
You can figure basic water amounts at one gallon per person per day. This would be enough to drink and cook with but only leaves a minimal amount with which to wash up. Some ideas to help out here are to stock up on wet-wipes, hand sanitizer, paper plates and so on. Water need not be purchased for storage. Just rinse out old two-liter soda bottles and fill with tap water. Store them in a dark closet because sunlight could cause algae to grow.

19

Food

What kinds of food should one store? For the basic three week supply you should consider foods that are already prepared or that require minimum preparation. Plan on preparing and eating these meals in the absence of water and electricity. Pop Tarts, granola bars, cans of fruit and fruit juice boxes all work just fine for breakfasts. Canned soups, ravioli, tuna, canned ham, peanut butter, jelly, and crackers and such foods work fine for heavier meals. If you have a camping stove and adequate fuel it is simple to cook up ramen noodles, rice, heat up water for coffee and tea and so on. Throw in some "comfort foods" such as your favorite candy bars and the like. The bottom line is you want foods that store well and are easy to prepare and clean up after. To keep your food fresh (a relative term we have discovered) and avoid the strain of eating "strange foods" you should consider buying foods you normally eat. This way rotating your stock is simple - eat the old stuff first.

Hygiene

Remember to include sanitary supplies, soap, toilet paper and so on - you really do not want to run out of these types of things when you already have enough problems to deal with. Think about what you will do for a toilet if yours no longer works. At any rate, you'll want to consider sanitation and have basic supplies on hand. This includes diapers and wipes if you have infants

Medications

Ensure you maintain an adequate supply of any needed medications. You do not want to get caught in some kind of emergency with only two days of your daily medications left in the bottle. If you have little ones think about fever medication also. We have found that liquid Motrin works very well on our children. Have a good first aid kit in the home - keep it up to date. You should also have basic medical skills in the form of first aid and CPR training. People are injured every day and every day citizens respond by saving lives using rudimentary medical skills. Unfortunately, every day people also die because no one on the scene has these vital skills. The basic Red Cross first aid course can be completed on a single Saturday. Give them a call.

If you wear glasses or contact lenses you will need to provide spares here as well as any needed solutions and cases. If you or someone in your family uses hearing aids you will need to account for these and batteries as well.

Equipment

There are some other basics you need to have. Flashlights and spare batteries will be needed in most kinds of emergencies. Every member of our family has a flashlight next to their bed. Maglites are great value for the money and also make excellent gifts anytime. You should keep one in your car also. A portable radio and spare batteries could mean a great deal when it's your only form of contact with official information. NOAA weather radios are a nice addition as well. You will need basic tools like a hammer and saw, and a wrench to turn off your gas in the event of an earthquake. Know where your gas shut of is and how to turn it off. Once you turn it off you need to let the utility company turn it back on. This is a safety thing – they will inspect for leaks first to ensure you don't have an explosion. Having some plastic sheeting or tarps and duct tape and nails on hand would be nice if you had to make quickie repairs to a window or roof damaged in an emergency.

Information

Additionally, you will want to prepare an information packet. One item in it is a family contact plan. If an emergency occurs while you are at work and the kids are at school you will want a card in your wallet or purse with vital phone numbers. You children should have a card with these numbers also. Go ahead and plug the numbers into your cell phones if you own them – but also do the card. Your phone could stop working for a variety of reasons.

Everyone should also have the name and number of an out of state contact – say Aunt Millie. Many times in an emergency, local lines are overwhelmed but long distance lines remain open. In this case, Aunt Millie could act as a relay for information from the family as members call in from different locations. We are talking about land lines here. Cells almost always get overwhelmed in emergencies and cell phones no longer work.

You should have a list posted of important numbers – fire, ambulance, police, etc. If 911 is overwhelmed but you know the actual number to the local station, that could be helpful. Same goes for doctors, insurance companies and so on. Don't forget neighbors and relatives.

You will want some spare cash and coins. Keep the denominations small – vendors will not feel like making change in an emergency. Also keep Xeroxed copies of your credit cards and a list of bank account numbers. Include any other important documents like driver's licenses, leases, wills and so on. It would be a good idea make an inventory of your personal belongings and maintain that for insurance purposes also.

Remember to include copies of prescriptions for medicines, glasses and so on. A set of maps of the area are nice to have to keep track of what you are hearing over the radio.

All of this information could be placed on a memory stick but you should also have paper back up copies.

Evacuation Kit (72 Hour kit)
An emergency could arise that would force you and your family to rapidly evacuate your home. You should have sub-kits made up that contain additional basics such as a change of clothing, important papers, perhaps some cash and of course, food, water and basic first aid equipment. These kits should be easy to access on the way out of the home and should be sized so that they are easy to carry to the vehicle. A suggested list of items to include in your Evacuation Kit it is located at Appendix C.

The above food, water, medical items, gear and information are just the bare minimums. Having sufficient stocks of these items on hand does not make one a survivalist - not even close. They just make you a good citizen. In the aftermath of an emergency it takes time for the wheels of government to start turning and aid and assistance to start flowing. This is why our government would like to see every citizen take these simple basic steps. If you have taken care of the basics an emergency need not be a crisis.

These items, skills and more will be covered in more detail later but before you can go much further you will have to have the cooperation of your significant other.

Getting the Spouse on Board

I am going to assume that one of the adults in the family is convicted to prepare for potential future emergencies and, as is many times the case, the other spouse is "less than enthusiastic". A majority of the time it is the male that takes the lead in preparing while the female resists. This does not always hold true however.

I had a female friend who was (and still is) very active in the survivalist movement - much to the displeasure of her husband. "Mrs. Brown" was active on the internet, organized group events, and went out of her way to educate other survivalists. She became a major player in some circles and I think her husband resented it. He should have embraced it.

As I said though, usually it is the male who wants to prepare while his partner is dragged kicking and screaming - if at all - into the survivalist mindset. Why is this?

Warning: I am about to get "politically incorrect" and/ or "sexist". It is not the first time and it will not be the last – you have been warned.

Roles

Generally speaking, men are stronger and more aggressive than women. This is because they are designed by God or nature (take your pick - I'm not trying to offend you here) to be the Protector-Provider. Men are more apt to take action alone and of their own accord.

Women, on the other hand, are designed to Nurture. They raise and teach children so that society can continue. They keep the home front. They crave security and like to work in groups. How many men go to the restroom together as opposed to women? Okay, show of hands - who just threw the book across the room? Hey, these have been traditional roles for men and women in many societies and they existed for a reason. I'll admit, they may seem "out of step" with modern American society. That does not mean they are "wrong". Does this mean that women can't protect or provide? On the contrary. Want to see ferocity? Mess with a woman's children.

But herein lays the source of many of the problems: Men see the danger and want to take steps to mitigate it - thus they begin preparing. Women, who crave security, do not want to be confronted with the idea of fighting for survival in some end of the world scenario and so reject all actions associated with it.

What to do?

The first and most vital step is communication. You must be able to talk to your spouse. To get them to participate you must first ensure they understand your thinking. If you are a man, you must convince your wife without scaring her. If you are a woman, you must convince your husband without making him think you are usurping his role of protector/provider. Scare the woman or threaten the man's position and you are in for a tough time.

Communication, trust, and honesty are key ingredients to a successful relationship. You have to be able to *talk* to your loved one. Try it. Turn off the television and computer for a week. Spend time talking. It is amazing how little real communication goes on between couples these days. My wife and I got disgusted with television once and just gave both of them away. For the first week we went through withdrawal. This was before we had computers and were hooked up to the Internet. We just didn't know what to *do* after we put the kids to bed and before we retired for the evening. Eventually, we started talking again. Our children started reading. We started remembering why we fell in love in the first place. It was a joy to spend time together. A few years later we bought another television but we go through periods of time where we box it up and stash it in the basement.

An amusing aside - I once saw a bumper sticker on a car that said, "Kill your TV". The driver had parked it outside of a video rental store and was dropping off movies! His TV was obviously not quite dead.

Phrasing
Instead of telling your wife you need to buy a year's supply of food to enable the family to survive the aftermath of a nuclear holocaust (which is very scary), try expressing it in terms of how convenient it will be if you don't have to run out for food right before the next big snow storm. Couch it in terms of basic economics - if you buy an entire case of tuna when it

goes on sale instead of just three or four cans you will experience significant overall savings.

Instead of telling your husband you have found a survivalist group and are going to prepare for Armageddon with or without him, discuss possibilities with him and ask "what if?" questions. Lead him to the conclusion that in order to "protect and provide" you both need to work on some additional areas of your life.

Baby Steps

Once the subject of preparing is broached, you should resist the urge to try and get your spouse totally involved all at once. It probably won't go very well if your first major conversation on survivalism begins with something like, "Honey, I think we should buy a three year supply of food, an arsenal of weapons, and 200 acres of land for a survival retreat." Baby steps are called for. Approach things slowly - ease into it.

Let's take camping. The ability to camp comfortably is an important survivalist skill. The first time my wife and I camped together was in the backpacking course I wrote of earlier. We were both young college students and it was only for one night. The next time was five years and a child later. My wife was not too enthused about heading off into the woods with an eleven month old baby for the weekend. The way she saw it, she had her hands full with the normal chores and keeping up with the baby in a clean, well lit environment with hot running water. Trying to do all that in the woods didn't seem like a good time to her. My goal was first, to convince her to go and second, to make her enjoy it to the point that she wanted to go again. The thing

I did *not* want to do was to create an event where she would forever say, "I tried it once and it was terrible - never again!"

I resolved to make it as much like an enjoyable break from her day to day routine as possible. I did everything. I planned the route to the national forest. I shopped for the food. I packed the car. I took everything I could think of to ensure she was comfortable - chairs, coolers, changes of clothes, plenty of cold drinks. When we got there I unloaded the car, set up the tent, built the fire, cooked the food, and so on. I suggested she take our son down to the small creek to play. I cooked and served the food, cleaned up afterwards - the works. She had a wonderful time. We have since made camping a family activity and everyone pitches in. Setting the stage was important though. If I had convinced her to go on a campout where we "roughed it" the first time we would probably have never camped again.

At this point some of you are thinking, "My spouse considers a hotel with no room service roughing it". That's okay - work with what you have. You may have to start out having picnics at a park before you can even begin to think of getting your loved one to spend the night in the woods. If that's what it takes, that's what it takes. Baby steps.

Shooting

Let's look at another activity where men routinely mess up where their wives or girlfriends are concerned: shooting. I did it - out of ignorance. I was back from college for a summer hanging out with my buddies and we decided to go shooting. My girlfriend tagged along. We ended up shooting skeet from a hand thrower with twelve gauge 00 Buck. For those who don't know, this is a weapon/round combination that produces significant recoil. It's also not the correct round for shooting clay pigeons but that's all we had with us at the time. Kids.

My girlfriend had never fired a gun before and wasn't too interested in shooting this day. I pestered her until she tried. The gun kicked, she missed, my buddies laughed. She hated it. It is a testament to her grit and determination that she overcame my stupidity and went on to become quite a shooter, attending several shooting schools and courses and instructing other women how to shoot. She also uses this experience as an example of what *not* to do.

Guys, don't try to "get the little lady to shoot the .44 Magnum" first time out. This is stupid. Start small and build. If you want your wife or girlfriend to shoot - consider hiring a female instructor. Men have ego, testosterone and such that can interfere with teaching women. Of course this does not apply to all men nor does it apply to all women.

My wife instructed one woman who was deathly afraid of firearms. Her husband wanted her to learn and so hired my wife. The class started with a couple of hours around a kitchen table - not on the range. By the time they got to the range, the student was still afraid but determined - she had a lot of "baggage" in her past she needed to work out. When she fired her weapon the first time, she cried. My wife continued to work with her. This woman has since become a skilled hunter who regularly takes grouse, deer and bear in the Oregon woods. Baby steps.

Money

Another thing to consider is money. Let's face it - we are not all millionaires who can buy whatever we like. For that matter, most millionaires can't buy whatever *they* like. You cannot expect a lot of success if you look at your not-quite-on-board spouse and say, "let's spend the next six months' salary on survival goodies." Again, you will have to go slow. Communication is going to be important here again. Start off with little things. Explain why you need them. Come to some consensus. If you must sacrifice something to buy some needed supplies, try to make the sacrifice from your end. Give up that fishing trip before you tell her to quit buying expensive baskets or vice versa if it's the other way around. Eventually it will work out and you will both agree on priorities. We are talking about the beginning stages here though - you want this to work out in the short term to ensure long term success.

I have a friend who saw the need to prepare and built a pantry in his house. His wife thought it was silly but went along with it. Then came the time when he wanted to stock it. She saw no reason to keep that much food on hand. She did not want him to go out and buy enough food to fill it up. So he did it slowly. She normally did the shopping and he helped her arrange food in the new room as she brought it home. Once a week for a month or so though, he would stop by the grocery store on the way home from work and announce upon entering the house that he had "just picked up a couple things". It worked for awhile. Then his wife noticed the shelves filling up and put her foot down again. Until one day when she needed some cream of mushroom soup for a casserole she was preparing and remembered that she had forgotten to get some after she used the one can she normally kept on hand. My friend calmly went into the pantry and returned with a can he had purchased earlier. Did he gloat? Did he rub it in her face? Indeed, no. He merely pointed out very gently that *that* was one of the nice things about having a pantry. She was sold. Baby steps.

Threat-based Planning

You've done your bit - you have communicated, shared your thoughts and concerns and brought your spouse slowly along until he or she is firmly on board. You have taken care of the basics as outlined previously.

Congratulations! You are now a team. But you still have much to do.

Before you get into serious preparing you need decide just what you are preparing for and design a plan that provides for a systematic approach. Failure to do so could be expensive at best and futile at worst. You must do some Threat-based Planning.

Threat Identification
The first step is to identify potential threats to you and yours. Get out a pencil and pad of paper, pour a couple cups of coffee (or whatever) and have a family meeting. Historically, what are the most likely threats in your area? If you live in Florida, it may be hurricanes; in Kansas it would be tornados and

possibly winter storms; parts of California are at risk for forest fires, earthquakes, mud slides and so on.

Having looked at those types of natural threats, you now should consider things like nuclear power plants to your west and north (generally upwind). Look at railroads and major highways in your area - chemical spills can be nasty. Do you live in an area where the threat of terrorism is very real? If so, write those down as well. Are you at risk of losing your job due to the changing economy? If so, this is a threat to your family's well being and must be included. Do you think a major strike or other shutdown of something like the trucking industry is possible? If so, this is something you want to consider as well. Nuclear war? Comet strike? UFOs? It's only silly if you think it doesn't apply to you. If it's something you are concerned about then it is real. Think through and write down every possible threat that could affect you.

Threat Assessment
Next, you need to rank order all of these threats. Do it two ways: first by likelihood of occurrence and second by magnitude of effect. For example, if you live in upstate New York the likelihood of a major winter storm is high and it goes to the top of your list. You may assess the likelihood of nuclear war as low but its effects as catastrophic so it would rank high on your "magnitude of effect" list.

Now comes the subjective part - you must combine the two lists into one using your judgment and best guesses. You will rank order your threats from greatest to least.

If you perceive your greatest threat is a potential ice storm which knocks out power and services for two weeks then you will need to prepare for two weeks of dealing with a cold, dark house and closed grocery stores. If you believe your greatest threat could be thermonuclear war and its aftermath then you have significantly more to prepare for. I don't have the answers for you – you will have to do your own assessment.

Once complete, you will have your own personal list of threats. Based on your threat list you will now be able to set priorities for your journey deeper into survivalism.

Task List

You will next identify and prioritize tasks. "Prepare" is a verb and you are going to prepare. You must complete tasks. These can be either mental or physical. For our purposes, spiritual tasks fall under the mental category. Mental tasks include planning, learning a new skill, deciding on a course of action and so on. Physical tasks include building things, buying supplies, organizing items and so on. Most tasks require that you expend mental energy before you get to work on the physical side.

Perhaps one of your tasks is to learn more about a particular threat – say nuclear war. That would be a good idea because you will not be able to make sound decisions without some knowledge base. Maybe you want to research nuclear power plants in your area to see if any are up wind.

As I said earlier, certain basics apply across the entire spectrum of emergencies. You will need shelter, food, water, sanitation, medical supplies and so on. Providing for these basics might be a good thing to put high on the list of tasks.

Soon you will have so many individual tasks written down that you may begin to feel overwhelmed. Do not despair! You are now going to make a Plan. In fact, you are going to make three plans: short term, mid-range and long-range plans.

Plans

Your short term plan should look out three or four months. These are things you want to do right now – secure a water supply, extend your prescriptions, get that dental work done, and so on. Go ahead and schedule these tasks on a calendar. Select the day(s) you are going to perform these tasks and get to it.

Mid-range planning will take you from four months out to a year or eighteen months in the future. Perhaps you need to wait until spring to put in that garden; or maybe you won't secure that supply of firewood until fall. Perhaps you simply have too many more important tasks to complete before you get those of lesser importance. Your mid-range plan should be in the form of a list of tasks assigned to specific months in the future.

It is important to actually choose dates – actual days in the case of your short range plan and months for your mid-range plan. This type of organization will help to ensure you do not procrastinate. Put the effort into this planning and then commit!

Finally, we come to long range planning. This is for any task you want to do but not in the next eighteen months. This could include tasks for which you do not currently have the resources to complete. Resources usually fall into one of two categories: Time or Money. Maybe you plan on moving to a different location, or building a new home or something similar. Perhaps it is just a task that needs to be done but you also have lots of other, more important tasks which must be completed first. At any rate, go ahead and make a list of these long range plans and organize it by year.

Do not get upset when your plans change. They will. You will find that life will interfere with your schedule, or you will develop new priorities and so on. That's ok – at least you now have a basis for accomplishing tasks. You should probably pull your plans out and look at them at least every other month or so. You will need to do this to schedule formerly mid-range tasks onto your short range calendar and to monitor your overall progress. Once a year you should go through the entire set of plans and readjust as needed.

Skill sets, Sharing

As part of your planning, you should have identified desirable skill sets – things you and your family need to know and be able to do. Some you may already have mastered – if one of you is a nurse for instance, then home healthcare should be taken care of. Others will have to be learned. Perhaps you determine someone in the family must learn about growing vegetables, or learn how to fix broken down engines. Let's face it – in any kind of emergency you will have to do things you don't typically do – you will have to take emergency action. What those things are depends entirely on the emergency. It could be as mundane as stapling plastic over a broken window to setting a broken leg – it all depends on what situation you end up in. That's why you did a threat assessment.

You should try and divvy up the various skills to be learned to every member in the household. At first it will be easy since we all fulfill certain roles anyway. The cook may be the one to learn how to cook with wheat for instance. Others will just have to be negotiated.

> *A human being should be able to change a diaper, plan an invasion, butcher a hog, conn a ship, design a building, write a sonnet, balance accounts, build a wall, set a bone, comfort the dying, take orders, give orders, cooperate, act alone, solve equations, analyze a new problem, pitch manure, program a computer, cook a tasty meal, fight efficiently, die gallantly. Specialization is for insects. – Robert A. Heinlein*

Full blown survivalists families will seek to have at least a working knowledge of as many self-sufficiency skills as possible. Despite Heinlein's quote to the contrary, people *should* specialize in certain tasks. Instead of having one person learn four new tasks, have every member of the family learn a different one very well. Doing so allows the family to cover a much broader spectrum of skills with some type of useable depth.

In our family, my wife handles food and animal husbandry. She researches various food storage options, procures food and manages the inventory. She practices new ways to cook outdoors and practices various means of food storage. She also sees to raising and caring for the dogs, chickens, goats and horse. She has developed some veterinarian skills, some leatherworking skills (horse tack) and so on. She is also a firearms instructor and sees to training the children as well as friends in basic gun safety and handling. She has many more skills but that provides an example.

Now, if I also tried to learn as much as she knows about food and critters, I would have less time to work on developing skills in carpentry, engine repair and so on. Does this mean I know nothing about taking care of animals or that my wife knows nothing about working on cars? To the contrary – we each teach the other various aspects of our "specialty". This is referred to in other circles as "cross training". It takes a specialist (to one degree or another) to cross train others. It does no good for your family if only one person knows everything there is to know about a subject – if something were to happen to that member, the family would lose an entire skill set.

Another point – just because a person is the "specialist" in an area does not mean that person does all of the related work. My wife does not do all of the food work or animal work – she supervises it. We all pitch in to help. This is a form of cross training by osmosis.

With children, you have more responsibilities and more options. Children need chores to help them learn responsibility. You need extra help. Try and fit the chore to the child's ability and interest level. Our son wants to be a doctor – guess who is primarily responsible for helping mom with medical matters? Home schooling and assigning specialties go hand in hand. Let your child study up on a particular area, give him or her responsibility and watch them grow!

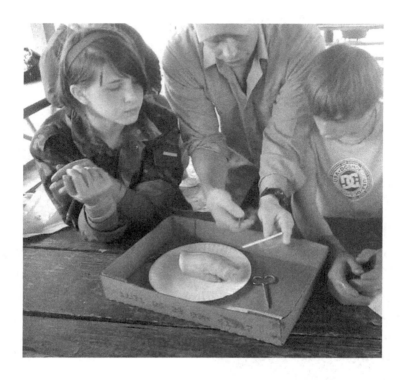

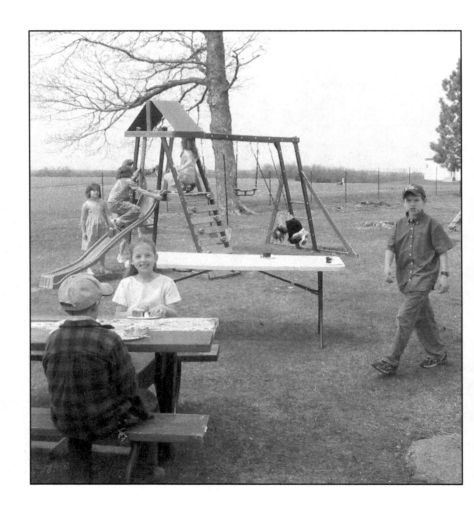

"It's for the Children"

This part of the book is for those of you with or who plan on having children. It will address skills you may want to ensure your children obtain. When imparting these skills it is important that you tailor the instruction to your child's maturity level and attention span. Keep it fun - childhood is supposed to be a fun learning experience not boot camp.

Kids and Camping

Getting the kids away from the constant stimulation of TV, Nintendo, CDs, Toys, etc. and out into the woods where they can immerse themselves in the sights, sounds, smells, and feel of the REAL world will reap huge rewards for your little ones. You want to let them explore their world but you don't want them to get seriously injured, lost, etc. You also want to make camping (and outdoor adventures in general) a positive experience which they will want to pass along to your grandkids. Camping as a family is a great way to grow closer and to build, maintain and learn new skills applicable to a survival situation. With that in mind the following are some ideas you may want to try on family campouts.

Rules

Yes, rules. Kids need boundaries and these should be established immediately upon arrival. They can be modified as necessary.

Have kids carry their survival supplies from this point forward. (We will discuss those supplies in detail a bit further on.) Accidents/emergencies never happen when you think they will.

Everyone should pitch in to unload and set up camp. You want them to learn about teamwork and the importance of discipline in the wilderness. Give kids tasks they can do fairly easily - make it fun. Establish the perimeter. "You kids can play on this side of that big tree, over to that fallen log, over to the car bumper and back to the tree." The size of the perimeter will vary based on the area, the kid's abilities/maturity, etc.

Announce speed limits. We don't let our kids run inside the area bounded by the tents, fire, and "kitchen". We don't want them tripping over tent stakes, falling in the fire or knocking food into the dirt. We also don't let them run in the dark. They are usually getting tired and clumsy by then and we don't want them tripping on a rock and bonking their head.

Activities
You won't need a "training schedule" for your kids' time but you should have some things in mind that you would like to accomplish with them. We all keep busy schedules with work, getting meals ready, kids to school, sports, and so on. Take time to relax and let things flow a bit.

Camp set up
Children should be taught how to put up the tent(s). This doesn't have to happen the first time, nor all at once. If you merely have them "hold this" or "bring

me that pole", they will eventually get it. If they have their own "kids' tent" you should give them a class on setting it up and supervise them the first few times.

Fire building
Everyone should know how to build and use a safe fire. Have the kids help gather wood. Explain and have them help prepare a safe fire area. Show them how, and when they are ready- have them light the fire. Have them help maintain it. Finally, show and have them help put the fire OUT when you are finished.

Cooking
Knowing how to prepare good meals over a fire/in the outdoors is a skill all survivalists should have. Have the kids help with every meal. Try new things yourself every once and awhile. For lunch we usually just do sandwiches and juice but the kids help there as well. We keep fluids available at all times and push the kids to drink and unlike at home, we keep snacks fairly available too. Kids will be burning up a lot of energy and will need replacement. Try to keep it healthy.

Cleanup/Hygiene
Have them help. Teach them how to live comfortably in the woods. If you are in a camp ground with facilities you will of course use them. If you are in the outback you will have to construct a latrine, set your kitchen up for dishwashing, maintain personal cleanliness, haul water, etc. All this is "taught" by doing.

Teach a "class"
I usually try to teach at least one class to my kids and then have them perform the task. Things we have done in the past include shelter construction (lean to, debris

hut, wickiup) traps/snares; basic compass work; lashing, etc. When they actually perform the task they gain confidence as well as knowledge.

Nature observation/hike
It sounds like a given but observation can be guided to enhance kids' abilities. Take a slow hike. Let the kids range out a bit. Find/identify animal sign, find water, identify plants (eat some), look at "cool" rocks, sticks, etc. We like to camp near little (like 2 feet across) streams and let the kids play in/near them. This will occupy them for hours. Let them climb rocks, swing on vines, throw rocks, etc.

Toys
Ok we bring a FEW toys. If it's too hot, the kids are too tired or whatever, we let them spread out a blanket and play Barbie, Legos, etc. We control when and it is not much but if you are camping for a week or so the kids will appreciate it. Books are good too (especially if it is raining).

Sleeping
Make sure the kids are comfortable (warm/cool/bug-free enough). We let them use their pillows and we let them bring a stuffed animal if they want. When they were small they slept in mom and dad's tent. Now they have their own. At first we set their tent up so that we could see it from inside our tent. Now they want a little "space". We hang a kerosene lantern turned down low so they can be oriented if they have to get up in the night. When they were young we escorted them to the latrine at night. They are usually so tired that they fall asleep very quickly once we put them down.

Things to bring

Here are some things you might not normally think of to bring with kids along.

Extra clothing
You will want lots of extra clothes and a clothes line/ pins. If there is water or dirt your kids will find it. That's GREAT! What's not great is a shivering, filthy child for days on end.

Play pen
A play pen can be very useful for toddlers and below. Hey, sometimes you will have to take your eyes off Junior to get supper ready.

Diaper wipes
They are not just for babies – these wipes work great on bigger kids too for cleaning faces and such. They aren't bad for a quick "shower" for adults when nothing else is available.

Dining Fly
Dining flies or a tarp are great over a picnic table if it's raining and they give the kids someplace other than the tent to hang out.

First aid kit
You will want something bigger than the normal run-of-the-mill kit. You'll want one with a thermometer, children's Motrin, cold medicine, etc. Make sure you have supplies to deal with a gash (you may need more than a Band-Aid).

Towels

You can have the kids take sponge baths or you can make a tub. We did this once by using half of a large dog kennel with a tarp inside and overlapping. We poured cold water in it and heated it up with water from the kettle. You could also line a depression or hole with the tarp as well. My wife appreciated the bath after about a week in the woods!

If you haven't camped as a family you are missing out! If you are not familiar with camping, you should start. It doesn't take much money (don't let the gear catalogues fool you). It can be as simple as a Saturday-Sunday trip for which you cook hot dogs, make sandwiches and eat cereal. You may be restricted to camping close to your vehicle for awhile but that's ok too. Just get out there. Have fun!

Basic and Intermediate Skills for Children

Fitness

First your child must be physically fit. I'm not talking about being a tri-athlete but if he/she is fat, gets out of breath running across the back yard, or can't take a walk in the woods - that is YOUR fault. If that is the case - kill your TV, throw out the Nintendo, quit letting them eat marshmallows, etc. Those are just for starters.

You may want to look into organized sports as another option. Participating will teach your child team work, discipline, reward for effort, how to lose gracefully, and what it feels like to win. Swimming and soccer are excellent sports to increase endurance which is a key component of "survival fitness".

Make sure your children have a proper diet (as opposed to dieting). You know – meat, fruits, vegetables, wholesome foods. Avoid wasted calories like sodas, chips, candy and so on. I did not say eliminate them totally – just avoid them in general.

Take family walks after dinner - it promotes unity and burns calories. Making this a regular part of your day will allow your family to draw closer together. It not only promotes physical health, but also emotional health – you will actually talk to each other. You can point out interesting things, or bring up interesting ideas for your children to ponder.

You could take hikes on weekends – I'm not talking about death marches here but go ahead and pack a lunch. It's worth an hour drive to go someplace interesting to hike. It could be a state forest trail or a historical site or any of a number of interesting places. Try to avoid counting mall shopping as hiking.

We moved around a lot when our children were younger but everywhere we lived we hung a knotted rope up in a tree in the back yard. My kids learned to climb at early ages. It used to amuse me to see my young, skinny, little girl challenge much larger and older boys to climb the fifteen foot rope up to the branch. They would try and fail and then she would scamper up. Here is self-esteem!

Activities

Ok, now that our kids are in decent shape, what can we do to improve their ability in the survivalist arena? Start with their BOBs. I address BOBs later but I'd like to add a bit here as well. First, after you decide what it will contain, have your child help pack his/her BOB. They need to learn how to use everything in their personal pack. Not necessarily all at once, but it makes for nice Saturday activities to practice some of it a bit at a time (on that weekend hike maybe?)

When packing their clothes consider packing 'civilian' clothes instead of BDUs. Kids generally don't arouse a lot of suspicion in normal day to day activities, but a kid in BDUs will. For this reason it is best to just consider earth-toned civilian clothes. This is what I call "camo camo". Normal earth toned clothing will conceal the wearer in woods and fields if necessary but also works in more civilized settings. Wearing BDUs while shopping is not a good way to be "camouflaged".

Hiking and camping are wonderful activities for children. They are out in nature, away from the idiot box and they are learning survival skills by osmosis. Before you take your child to the woods you should ensure he/she has been given a lost-proofing class and has basic survival supplies. This would be a great activity for the first trip.

Two other skill areas children should be trained in include Lost Proofing and the Seven Survival Skill Sets. We will cover these in the next two chapters.

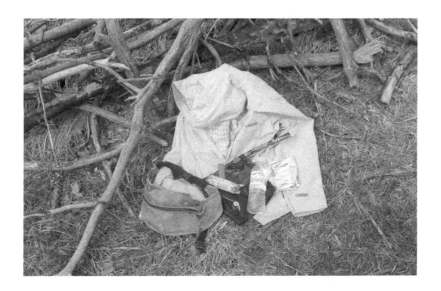

Lost Proofing

Children get lost in the woods every year. Many
had parents who cared and were trying to be "good
parents". Stuff happens. *If* it does, you want your
child to pull through.

The first thing you want to do is to prevent them
from getting lost. This is done by setting boundaries,
checking up on them frequently and so on. Your
children will have to be disciplined enough to obey you
when you say, "Don't cross the road" or "Don't go past
that big rock". This is not a book on child rearing so
you're on your own here.

Your children must be told that once they realize
they are lost, or once it gets dark and they are still
not back, they must - STOP. You don't want them
wandering farther away or off a cliff or into a sharp
stick. They should find a sheltered place and sit

49

down. I teach kids that after they sit down in a safe place they should empty their pockets. This gives them something constructive to do, keeps them from moving, and may help them to remember something they had that they would have otherwise forgotten.

Now, while they are stopped they could use some things to help them out. This is not a BOB. You cannot have a 4 year old girl constantly carrying around 5 lbs of equipment. It does no good to have a kid haul something around that you haven't taught him or her to properly use. (such as a lighter or matches). First, have your kids dress appropriately for the *potential* weather/environment. During Spring, showers can pop up unexpectedly and temperatures can rapidly drop. Just because it's warm now does not mean that Sally might not need a jacket later – especially if she has wandered away from you. Have her tie it around her waist. Some other stuff to consider:

Whistle
Have them wear it tucked in their shirt so it does not snag (enforce this rule). If the child is very young, put it on a piece of string that would break before choking the child. You don't want the child sliding down a steep hill and getting the necklace caught on some root and choking her. When you first start doing this with your kids have them blow it three times loud. This removes the curiosity and teaches them how to use it. Three of anything (whistle blasts, gun shots, smoke plumes) is the international signal of distress. Tell them it is *only* to be used if they are lost or hurt (enforce this rule vigorously) tell them "the boy who cried wolf" story. Tell them if they are lost to blow it three times every couple minutes. When they blow

their whistle, they should place their fingers in their ears. Some whistles are very loud and could hurt their ears. Either way, by plugging their ears when signaling and the child will be better able to hear a response.

Bright clothing or material

It is a whole lot easier to find a kid dressed in hunter orange than one dressed in BDUs. I also know that most of our kids wear "subdued" clothing in the woods. Have them carry a bright (I like orange) piece of material. Aluminum foil works also. Tell them if they are lost to put it on or spread it on the ground in front of them (not under the tree!). Cutting a hole in a large square of nylon/silky type cloth so they can slip it on like a poncho works well. Have them PRACTICE this - kids remember what they DO better than what they're told. If the child crawls up under a spruce tree or into a hollow log to get out of the weather, they have to make sure rescuers can see their signal if they happen by while the child is sleeping. Have them hang their signal head high and in a place where it can be seen from several directions.

Again, you have to practice this. You can make a game of it on hikes. "Where would you go right now if it was raining?" "
Where would you hang your signal?"
"Show me!"

Large trash bag

Cut a slit in the bottom for the head to poke out - Voila! instant poncho! (and it's warm too). Hypothermia is the biggest danger to lost kids. Ever see those large ORANGE trash bags on the side of the road??? (Get the picture?)

Light

I used to use chemical lights (a bit tough for a little child to activate though). One year for Christmas my children got those tiny l.e.d. lights - they put out a bright blue light that supposedly lasts forever. They are very small and weigh almost nothing. One good thing about chemical lights: I used to put an activated one on a string and make my kids carry them around at night while they were playing. It's tough to see children when they are outside of the campfire circle, and if one started wandering off or fell and became unconscious it would take a little while to find them without it. (My wife and I carry D-cell Maglites once it gets dark).

Snack

Your kids won't get fat snacking on a campout. Have them carry a granola bar, fruit roll-up, a pouch of those fruit-gel animals, or some such. It would be a good morale boost to a lost child to have something to chew on - plus it keeps them busy. A five year old could pull out an envelope of those fruit dinosaurs and play with them – passing time and taking their mind off of being lost.

OK, for a little kid we are now approaching the limits of what they can carry around all day. Some of the below items can easily be carried by larger/older children and/or kept in a small fanny pack for the little ones to carry when hiking with mom and dad or whatever.

Fluids

The best solution we have found is to consciously keep the kids hydrated during the day - that way if they get lost, they are starting with a "full tank". For carrying around you can use those little juice boxes with the straw or small bottled water for smaller kids- they are not going to carry a big canteen and have a good time. Larger children can carry water bottles, canteens, Camelbacks, and so on.

Space blanket
These work well and don't take up too much room. Again, have your kid PRACTICE with one by wrapping one around the top of the head and torso like in the picture on most of them.

The following items, if carried, are useful only if you have taught your child how to properly use them - some are even dangerous if they are used incorrectly.

Lighter/Matches/Tinder
Double wrapped in Ziploc back. Fine steel wool and dryer lint work well for tinder. So do Vaseline impregnated cotton balls. You can buy a little Ferrocerium rod and striker called a "Hot Spark" from Boy Scouts of America (it's available on the Internet.) These work well with the aforementioned cotton balls and in fact, my youngest daughter, starting at about age seven, started all her fires with one. She did not like using matches because she was afraid of getting burned.

First aid
Gauze, tape, Band-Aids, and so on can be used to keep a small injury from getting worse. It also allows the child to feel empowered – they are taking care of themselves.

Pocket knife
Make sure it's sharp. Make sure they know how to safely use one – we don't want them to have to use the first aid kit!

Cord
I like parachute or "550" cord – also known as "backwoods gold". It is very strong and has several smaller strings inside the outer sheath. Used for shelter construction, repairing stuff, etc.

Kids don't get lost when parents expect it. It's usually a case of, "I just turned around for a minute and he was gone!" That is why your child must have at least the basics to allow him/her to be found quickly. If you make the "kit" too large, the child won't have it when he needs it. They ARE kids, so you will have to check, re-check, reinforce, etc. Teach them how to use the gear, be positive (don't scare the little darlings - this is supposed to be fun!), and relax.....a bit.

Seven Survival Skill Sets

In addition to basic supplies, your children (and you too for that matter) need to have seven broad skill sets:

Water
Food
Shelter
Fire
First aid
Navigation
Signaling

All survival kits should cover these seven vital areas. In other words, all survival kits should contain items that allow you to use or procure items in those areas.

These are basic/intermediate skills. They are all fairly easy to learn but like everything else, to really learn them you must PRACTICE. This is especially true with kids - they remember what they DO. You do not have to do them all at once. In fact, children learn best in short doses with lots of hands on. Scouts will teach all of these skills to your children. I recommend you sign your child up and participate yourself as a parent - Scouting is a great organization. If you cannot join you can at least buy age appropriate books (Cub Scout manual, Boy Scout manual, etc) and work through the activities with your child.

WATER
Your child needs to understand the importance of proper hydration and how to procure and treat water. Streams, ponds, solar stills, rain - all are sources. Treatment includes boiling, purification tablets, filters, bleach.....and on. Let your child actually do these things - it is the only way they will remember.

FOOD
He/she also needs to know how to procure and prepare food. Things that come to mind are: wild plant identification; traps and snares; hunting; animal sign identification; how about opening a can with a pocket knife? They should know how to dispose of trash in a sanitary and secure manner. They should know which parts of the above plants are edible and how to prepare them. They should know how clean, butcher and cook critters. Teach them to cook at

home, let them do a little on campouts. Have them help clean up. Now obviously, your 15 year old daughter will be able to do much more than your 5 year old son - keep things at a level your child can handle.

SHELTER

Knowledge here will allow your child to stay warm or cool, dry and safe when circumstances are 'less than optimal'. Things that come to mind are: knowing how to set up a tent; poncho hooches, brush shelters, avoiding hypothermia, flash flood and lightning considerations, and on.... Training here can be as simple as talking about it on hikes "would you want to set up a shelter here? Why not?" Playing in the park, setting up tents/shelters in the back yard and of course camping are all good ways to practice this as well.

FIRE

Fire is our friend - it keeps us warm, cooks our food and can be used to signal for help. It can also be dangerous so we must learn proper safety considerations as well. Your child should be comfortable with fires. He/she should know several ways of starting them. This can be done in the back yard too – when I lived in suburbia we taught a group of scouts fire-building in the back yard in an unused portion of the garden. We kept them very small - just enough to learn how to light them. Again, kids learn by doing.

FIRST AID

The biggest medical danger to lost children is hypothermia. Your child should know how to prevent, recognize and treat this killer. He/she should know how to treat cuts, stings, sprains, fractures, shock. All scout manuals cover these skills - Cub scouts at a lower level than Boy scouts and the First Aid merit badge book being the most advanced. Teach to the level your child can handle.

NAVIGATION
First teach (it is NOT innate) your kids the concept of direction. It amazes me how many adults, not to mention kids, have no concept of North, South, East and West. "This river is flowing north, which side are we on?" Teach them how to use their compass (they DO have one, don't they?) and read a map. Have your kids help navigate on car trips. Practice as a family on those walks you take. Many parks have orienteering courses set up that you can "play" on.

SIGNALING
Cloth, mirrors, whistles, smoke, lights, images stamped out in snow or sand, etc. can all be used for effective signaling. Teach your child when it is appropriate to signal for help. Have them practice - kids learn by doing (I keep pointing this out because it is important).

OK, so those are the basic and intermediate skills your child should know. Time spent learning how to do these things is so much more valuable than time spent in front of the idiot box. Remember to keep it fun. It should seem like a treat, not a chore to learn these things. What? You don't know how to do all of these things? Well they say kids learn by doing, so do adults. Even more so, adults learn by TEACHING. Sounds strange, doesn't it? Try it. "It's for the children."

"We're TRAPPED!"

The following story relates to an adventure I had with Boy Scouts and I'd like to share it with you for some of the lessons you can derive from it.

So there I was......In a land far away (a third-world tropical "paradise") talking to another American friend of mine who just happened to be the Scoutmaster for a small Boy Scout troop located in said country. "So, Joe" says he, "You're an assistant Cub-master (Cub Scouts) right? Wanna go camping with the troop next weekend? We need two adults and my assistant can't make it."

Boy Scouts requires at least two adults on every sanctioned activity – a good rule me thinks. Needless to say, I jumped at the chance to hike up a jungle-covered mountain and camp for a couple days.

We departed early on a Friday morning via bus and arrived at our start point at the foot of a largish mountain around mid morning. There were about 20 boys ranging in age from 11 to 16. After making sure the driver would return on Monday morning to take us back, we put on our backpacks and headed up the mountain. We followed a nice trail along a swift stream that was perhaps 30 feet wide. The trail was steep and muddy and some of the boys had never carried a pack before so we took our time. When we approached the spot where we would camp about half way up the mountain we had to cross the stream. The water was knee to thigh deep on me and swift. The locals had rigged a hand line of questionable strength across the stream and some boys were "challenged" by the crossing. I appointed myself lifeguard and moved down stream with a rope. I had all the boys release their waist straps and loosen their shoulder straps so they could dump their packs if they fell. We all survived the crossing.

We reached our jungle "camp" around 1 p.m. and started setting up. Unless one is in second growth, the jungle doesn't have that much undergrowth - it's too dark in there. The boys cleared some ferns and set up tents - not very well I might add. They tried to place new, inexperienced scouts with older boys. I rigged up a hammock with a poncho over top - I really don't like the idea of sleeping on the ground in jungle. The first day was uneventful: I assisted the Scoutmaster in setting up some observation areas for the boys who were working on Environmental Science merit badge; we cooked dinner on stoves and went to sleep.

I had forgotten how LOUD the jungle was at night. Some of the young-uns didn't get much sleep as every cicada and peeper frog sounded like the "creature from the bog". The boys had mosquito netting on their tents but I had none. No problem. Right before bed, I put on a set of BDUs, socks, gloves and a hat. I sprayed myself liberally with insect repellent, wrapped up in my poncho liner (because of the temperature difference, it felt cold at night) and blissfully surrendered to sleep. Until around 2 a.m. when OUCH!! It felt like someone was poking a hot wire into my inner thigh!! I quickly reached down and, through my pants, squished what turned out to be a very large ant, which was happily munching on my flesh. I pulled a flashlight from my shirt pocket to see how this had happened as immediately discovered two things: my poncho liner was dangling down to the ground thus providing a ladder for the ant and there were THOUSANDS of inch-long ants moving in a wide column under my hammock. I could actually hear them. I remember wondering how in the heck I would get out of bed in the morning and being glad that I didn't have "use a tree" at the moment. I tucked my pants legs into my socks, rubbed the welt on my leg and went back to sleep. There was no sign of the ants come morning.

The next morning the Scoutmaster took ALL of the older, experienced scouts for a hike (Hiking merit badge) that was to last until mid afternoon. He left me with instructions to work on the Environmental Science merit badge with the young scouts; have them work together to make and eat lunch (soup and sandwiches); and gather wood for the evening's campfire. "No problem" says I, and off went the entire troop leadership.

The merit badge activities went fine. Lunch was OK but the boys did not work well together. Then IT happened. Suddenly. Violently. CRACK! BOOM! WOOOOOSH! A tropical thunderstorm the likes of which few Americans have experienced. They come without warning and the amount of water and wind is something to behold. The boys scattered to their tents. Since they had all set up with senior scouts, they were mostly all alone in their tents..... The tents started blowing down.... many boys started crying.... The storm was furious. I went running around and moved all of the boys into the only two tents that remained standing and then retreated to my hammock. The wind and lightning abated fairly quickly but it poured, and poured, and poured. The boys were miserable, wet huddled masses of humanity. They were having no fun.

I figured the storm would last an hour and then we could all get out and gather wood for that night's fire. The Scoutmaster had lugged a gallon of kerosene up the mountain so I knew we could get one started. The rain continued and I could not talk the boys out of their tents to help gather wood. They had ponchos but they were not going to play. "They need a morale boost - a paradigm shift," thinks I. So, I took off my shorts and shirt (don't worry, I was wearing running shorts underneath), put on my sandals, grabbed my soap and shampoo and walked into the middle of camp. It was raining harder than the water pressure of the shower in my house. I stood there, to the utter amazement of the youths and took a shower. "Come on out, the water's fine!" I shouted.

They went from morose to happy in seconds. Next thing I know, they are all out playing in the rain and helping to gather a large pile of wood. It stopped raining. Mid afternoon comes and goes.... no returning senior leadership. The happy mood is starting to slip as boys start to worry. One boy walks over to me and says, "Mr. Fox, there's a problem and I don't think they are coming back." He instantly has everyone's attention. "What's up?" says I. "Come look at the creek," says he. We all walked over the formerly swift 30 foot wide creek to see a 40 foot wide raging torrent of impassable river.

"We're TRAPPED!!!" screams one boy. Chaos ensues. Boys start crying again. They are moaning that we'd never escape, we're all gonna die, Yaada, Yaada,

Yaada. They are rapidly spinning out of control when I yell, "HEY!"

Silence. "Guys, what are you worried about? It's not raining; we have tents and ALL of the food! They are the ones who need to worry, not us! This water will go back down and we'll get out of here just fine." That worked pretty well but some then started grousing about what the other boys would do without tents, food, etc. I told them not to worry; the Scoutmaster would take care of them. And he did. Using that most essential of survival supplies (the credit card) he bought them dinner at a local eatery and put them up for the night in a local "motel". They loved camping that way.

I organized the boys for dinner, we pooled resources, reset up the rest of the tents, and went to bed at dark. The next morning, just as we were finishing breakfast, the Scoutmaster strolled back into camp with the older scouts. We had the campfire on Sunday night and all ended happily.

LESSONS LEARNED:

1. Boy Scouts is a great organization - get involved.

2. When crossing a tricky stream with rucks have a lifeguard with rope down stream, unbuckle waist straps and loosen shoulder straps.

3. Tuck your clothes in to avoid bugs - I'm sure that ant crawled up my pants leg from my foot. Don't let your poncho liner touch the ground!

4. Make sure tents are set up correctly the first time.

5. Think positively and deal with the environment - don't roll into a fetal position, suck your thumb and say, "oh poor, dear me..."

6. Flash flooding is a real danger in some parts - be aware of it.

7. Don't allow panic to spread - take charge and take action.

8. Be flexible, adapt, improvise.

9. "Don't leave home without it"

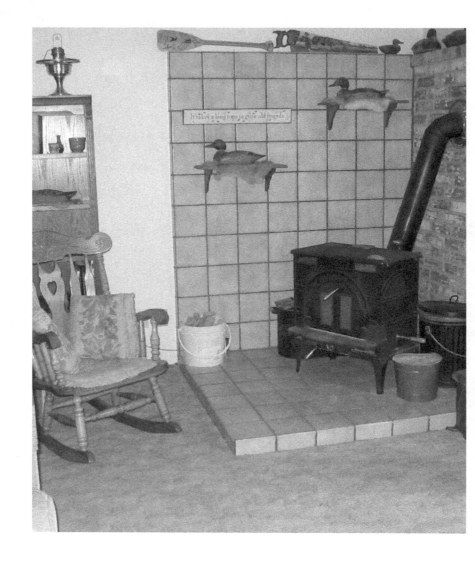

PUTTING IT ALL TOGETHER

Survival Budgeting

Preparing costs money. Everything costs money and for most of us this is a finite resource. You are going to have to put some thought into a budget for your family's preparedness.

Most Americans are in debt. Debt is bondage and you need to get out of it. First and foremost – stop buying stuff on credit if you cannot pay it off when the bill comes at the end of the month. My grandfather refused to buy anything on credit – including his house. Most of us cannot afford to pay for our home outright if we buy instead of rent but that may not be terrible. What is terrible is taking out second and third mortgages to pay for trifles. That's my opinion, anyway – if you want to ride the housing market bubble then go for it. *I wrote that last sentence in 2006 and I wish more people had had similar thoughts before that bubble burst.*

You will not be able to go out and in one month buy everything you need to survive your ultimate survival scenario. First you have to prioritize what you need. Just like in threat-based planning you need to rank order what you need. You may have to save a little bit every month until you are able to buy that piece of gear you've been wanting – that's ok, it will be worth the wait.

"How much is your life worth?" You are going to hear this more and more as you start considering various preparedness items for purchase. This is a trap you must avoid! See, Americans have this problem – they think they can solve problems by throwing more money at them. Instead of investing time and effort, we would rather buy the latest, greatest, "new and improved" version of something. We also want to keep up with the Joneses. Take golfers (I used to be one): they will go out and spend a couple hundred dollars *on one club* just "to get a few extra yards out of my drive". Or some bicyclist will spend good money on titanium forks "to shave a few ounces off of the bike". Both think spending money will improve their performance. It might.

I submit however that the golfer could have made better use of his money by taking a lesson or two and spending more time on the driving range with several buckets of balls. The bicyclist could have almost certainly shaved a few *pounds* from his body weight by eating less – never mind a few ounces from his forks (the bike doesn't roll down the road by itself after all). But spending the money on the latest doo-dads allows them to show off to their buddies, to fool themselves into thinking they don't have to put effort into improving, they can just purchase it.

Let's review some examples. You decide you want a largish knife to go in a survival kit you will keep in your vehicle at all times. You do research, you talk to knowledgeable friends; you shop around. Guess what? You can spend a few hundred dollars and buy the super-duper combat tested Warrior Tool. Oh yes, you will be able to read about this in knife magazines, on the Internet and your knife buddies will know all about it. You will say something like, "wow, that's a lot of money for a knife" and someone will reply with, "How much is your life worth?" Guess what? You can get very close to the same level of performance (because you are not really going to hack at concrete and steel with your survival blade, now are you?) with a two dollar carbon steel butcher knife you buy used at the local thrift store.

You may decide you need a rifle to hunt deer with. Maybe you even decide to put a scope on it. You could go buy a used but perfectly acceptable Remington 700 with a scope for a few hundred bucks at a gun show. Or, you could spend a couple thousand dollars for a "sniper rifle". Hey, what's your life worth?

Here is reality. I have trained many people to shoot. I have been around many more that shoot regularly. I am a good shot. Having established that background we come to this: Most people cannot shoot up to the level of their weapon. More simply put – for the vast majority of shooters the lowly standard grade bolt gun will shoot just as well as some accurized wonder rifle. Spend the extra money on other preparations.

You *should* make your survival preparations a priority though. Time could be short. What's more important – season tickets for the local professional football team, or setting up some kind of system to stay warm during the winter – without utilities? Could you give up eating out every now and then and use that money to increase your food storage? Sure you could. Just make a conscious decision to do so.

Family Activities

By choosing to become more prepared you will also find yourself favoring some types of activities over others. Take reading for example: you could read a trashy romance novel or the latest detective thriller, or you could read a book about how to perform home childbirth, or intensive gardening. You could spend every Sunday watching football after church or you could take hikes with your family. Would it be better to play a computer game or practice marksmanship? Watch a video or build a rabbit hutch?

My point is, with only so much free time, we have to consider how we use it. You might as well use it doing things which will make you and your family more prepared for what is undoubtedly coming down the pike.

One thing you should definitely consider is getting into better shape. When it's time for the family to go into "survival mode" you will all need to be strong. Remember the desire to spend money we spoke about earlier? Avoid it. It does not cost money to get into shape or lose weight. Not really.

Get Fit
If you need to lose weight forget diets. Just eat sensibly. If you don't know what sensible is – look it up on the Internet or discuss it with your doctor. Eat balanced meals, eat your veggies, eat normal portions, eat at least three times a day and cut all of the garbage out of your diet. Easy to write – harder to do. But you *can* do it.

Should you join a gym or invest in home exercise equipment? You could, but I advise against it. Start with family walks. If your little girl walks a lot slower than you – throw on a rucksack! Take jogs, do manual labor if you don't already – split your own firewood instead of paying someone to deliver it, carry feed sacks, move your water barrels. Do push ups and situps. Until you can do a hundred of each straight through, you probably do not need to worry about buying special equipment – there is progress to make right there on the living room floor!

Whatever you do, start out slow and build up gradually. If you are really out of shape, see a doctor first and discuss a workout program.

Get Outside

Learn to enjoy outdoor activities. If you and your family are ever thrown into a survival situation you will be spending a lot of time in the outdoors. The time to grow hardy is now! Join an orienteering club – you will learn to use a map and compass and get comfortable moving through the woods in all kinds of weather. You will learn about proper clothing and footwear and gain a lot of confidence.

Go camping. You need not spend a lot of money. All you need is tent and some blankets. If it's cold or if you want (I do) you can buy a sleeping pad for each family member for just a few bucks at Chinamart. Sure, you can spend more. Don't bother – especially at first. Start by camping in the back yard, progress to a local campground, then to a more remote campground. You will learn new things every time you go.

Camping too hard? Go on a picnic like we discussed above. Take Saturday walks with the whole family in the local park. Pack a lunch and take along a plant identification book. Have the kids look for animal tracks. Identify them too.

Get Educated

Go on field trips as a family. Most counties have a county fair every summer. You can learn a lot about livestock and raising crops by talking to people. Does your area have a museum? Go and learn how the Native Americans lived in your area. Learn what the local pioneers did to survive. Many times you can pick up tips that will work in your geographical region.

Pick a project such as making a candle lantern or baking bread and get the whole family involved. The wonderful thing about the Internet is that you can get instructions to do just about anything. The key is to actually do the activity though instead of just reading about it, or maybe printing off the instructions and filing them away "in case you ever need them". Nope, you will learn much more by doing. Go and Do.

Team Building – The Tight Family Unit

Whatever comes down the pike – you will face it as a family. Hopefully you have a strong team and you can operate synergistically as a unit. However, I understand that in this hectic, modern world it is tough to forge and strengthen family bonds – we are

all just so *busy.* Dad has a Rotary Club meeting or
is playing cards with the guys; Mom is attending a
work function or playing Bunko with her friends; the
kids have soccer practice, music practice, or they are
spending the night at a friend's or going to a movie
or... It's just tough to carve out time to be together.
So here are some suggestions to help your family
strengthen relationships now, in good times, so that in
times of trouble and stress you can pull through.

Eating Supper Together
Such a simple thing. So important. And yet –
something that is becoming a rarity in our go-go-go
world. There is something magical and spiritual
about breaking bread together. There is something
wonderful about sitting around a table, enjoying a
meal and talking about – *whatever!* I know family
time schedules are often out of synch. I know we are
busy. I still strongly recommend that if you are not
already doing so, that you make a strong commitment
to eat as many suppers together as possible. Sure – it
may mean a late supper. Or an early one. Just have
supper when everyone can be there. *Make* everyone be
there. And please – do not sit in front of a television
or computer. Don't focus on the news or a movie or a
game – focus on your spouse and kids. You'll be glad
you did.

Family Home Evening
The Church of Latter Day Saints (Mormons) has
this excellent concept/practice. One night a week is
carved out for the family to stay home together and
participate in a fun and useful activity. This is the
priority and nothing may interfere with it. It is a time
to focus on each other and on God. You do not have

to be a Mormon to do this!   Relationships – whether building them, strengthening them, or repairing them – require a commitment of time. This is one way to provide "quality time" for you and your loved ones. You can Google "family home evening" and discover many wonderful resources to help out in this area.

Family Worship
This book has been and is primarily about physical survival. But what is even more important is spiritual survival. What is even more important is not tomorrow or next week but eternity. I remember a bumper sticker from several decades past that said, "The Family That Prays Together – STAYS Together". There is a lot of truth in that.

As a SERE instructor in the military I read numerous accounts of, and therefore taught that survivors – those who make it through harrowing ordeals, frequently had one thing in common. They had *faith* in something bigger than themselves.

I encourage you to worship as a family. Frequently. Draw closer to God, as a family, and you will see wonderful things happen in your home.

Setting Up House

Finding Space
One thing you will notice as a budding survivalist is than in order to prepare for future emergencies you will need to accumulate "stuff". You will probably accumulate more "stuff" than your average neighbor.

You will have to figure out ways to store it, organize it and secure it.

What you decide to accumulate is entirely up to you and should derive from the *threat-based planning* you already did. I have included appendices to help guide you through several preparedness areas.

Most of us have some financial limitations – we cannot simply buy a bigger house to accommodate our new lifestyle choices. You will inevitably have to work with what you have. That's okay – the good news is you *can*.

Your initial problem is probably going to be finding storage space for all of your new goodies. Many kitchens are built nowadays with limited cupboard space and if they have a "pantry" at all, it is usually just a glorified broom closet with shelves. Storing weeks to months of extra food will require some additional space. The same goes for all of the other supplies you may end up procuring from tools to Band-Aids.

Finding "hidden" space becomes more important. There is space under couches and beds. You can increase the space by placing the furniture legs on blocks or bricks of some sort to increase the height even more. You can place dust ruffles along the bottom edges to hide what is beneath. Most closets have unused space above the shelf. Add a shelf above the existing one – go around three sides instead of just one.

Containers

You will want to keep your supplies safe from things
that can hurt them. Depending on the particular
item, these things could include water, moisture, heat,
freezing, bugs, rodents, light (yes, light will damage
some things – like water), and so on. Cardboard boxes
are really only suitable for temporary storage – when
damp or wet they fall apart, rodents will eventually
chew through them, they get soft and lose their shape,
and they don't really stack well over time. Fear not!
There is a solution to your problem.

As you accumulate more goods you will undoubtedly
become familiar with bins and buckets. Rubbermaid
has a made a fortune from survivalists who purchase
their "Roughneck" bins in quantity. They come in
various sizes and colors for easy organizing; they are
tough, and they are inexpensive. Five gallon plastic
buckets are even better in some ways because you
can usually get them for free. Ask around your local
grocery store deli or bakery section. They will usually
save them for you if you ask – make sure to ask them
to save the lids also.

The buckets will have to be cleaned out but this is
easy to do with warm water and Dawn dishwashing
detergent.

Initially, you will be able to set the bins and buckets
around unused space such as behind furniture or
disguised with a throw as a lamp stand, end table or
some such. After you get to the point where you have
twenty or more of these containers you will need to
give serious thought to organizing your "survival stuff"
and may want to start thinking about building shelves

for them. If you design the shelves right you can have very little wasted space and still have access to each individual bin.

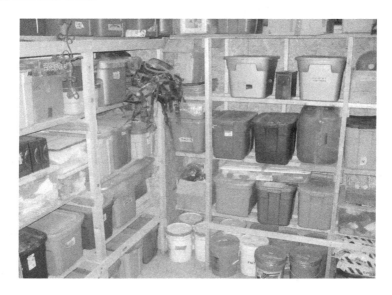

You may want to organize your gear by using different color bins. Put first aid supplies in red bins and camping supplies in green bins for instance. To know what is in each bin you will need to compile lists and label the outside of the containers. I used to just stick some masking tape on the outside of a bin and, using a permanent marker, write something like "camping supplies" or "candles" on the tape. There are two problems with this approach. First, anyone who sees your shelves (the neighbor borrowing your lawn mower, the plumber in for an emergency repair – whatever) will look at your nicely arranged containers and be able to quickly inventory your gear - not very security conscious of you. Secondly, that "permanent" marker will fade and the tape will come off leaving you with an unlabeled bin or bucket. Better to just number or letter your containers right onto the plastic. For example you can have bins 1 – 233 or buckets A – PP. Then you keep a list on a clipboard or in a binder that tells you what each container holds. You could have it broken down further by having a main index where you list the major type of supplies ("candles" or "socks") and then a separate set of lists that give detailed inventories of what exactly is in each container to include sizes, amounts and so on.

Organizing
Shelving is your friend. It does no good to have lots of great supplies if you cannot properly inventory and access it. When you need a water filter you will need to know where it is – stay organized. After you max out your basement and or garage you may find that you need still more space. This is where outbuildings come in. Sure, you could go down to your local home improvement place and buy a shed, but you'll learn a lot more if you build your own. It will be cheaper too – especially if you scrounge some materials. Yes, you CAN build it yourself. Do a little internet research, buy a book on basic carpentry, or ask a buddy to help. Who knows? Someday you may have to build a cabin.

So who is going to organize all of your gear and items? Who is going to manage it? It may end up being just you. A better solution is to have each family member take on certain responsibilities. In my family my wife handles the food (human, pet, and critter), medical supplies, and clothing. I handle the armory, camping supplies, and fuel. Generally speaking, try to let folks who handle related issues day to day handle the same preparedness issues.

Security

You are going to need to ensure you, your family, and your possessions remain safe and secure. Crime can be a problem now and it could potentially be disastrous after an emergency. The first thing you want to do is "maintain OPSEC" or operational security. Do not run around telling everybody in your neighborhood what you are up to. Do not show off your food storage, gun collection or anything else of value that someone may want to gossip about or steal. Instruct your children to do the same. Our kids have had standard instructions that if anyone asks personal questions such as, "what kind of guns does your daddy have?" they are to reply with, "my dad said for you to ask him." My child will then tell me about it as soon as possible.

Watch what you throw away. We live in the country so we can destroy old bills, check stubs and so on in a burn barrel. You may be able to do something similar or maybe you'll have to buy a shedder. Whatever you do, do not give personal information away. Be careful where you go and what you do on the Internet. I am no computer guru (but I have friends who are) so I won't give you anymore advice here except to say, get good firewall and antivirus software and learn how to use it.

Install good exterior doors and put deadbolts on all of them. If you have glass in or near the door you will need to use keyed deadbolts. The potential danger here is fire – keep the key in an easily accessible place but hidden from view near the door. Keep your door locked – whether you are gone or at home. Lock your windows. If you have windows open for ventilation figure out a way to "pin" them so they cannot be forced open wider. Many times you can drill through the window into the frame beneath and slip a long nail in there.

Install high intensity exterior lighting. Motion detector lights are very inexpensive and work well. You should install them to cover several angles of approach to your home or outbuildings. You may also want to install an alarm system. Basically, you will want some type of loud horn that goes off if someone breaks in (or you hit a panic button) and some type of system that lets you know if a door or window has been opened. You do not want to be surprised by someone sneaking up on or breaking into your home.

If you can have one, a good dog is a great asset. It does not even have to be a large dog (although we favor dogs in the "manstopper" weight class). A small, alert dog that yaps when strangers pull into the drive or walks towards the home is a good early warning system. Even better if you can have an outdoor dog and an indoor dog – the outdoor dog as an alarm and the indoor dog as a security protection device.

Domesticated fowl can be good roving alarm systems also. A flock of geese will raise a ruckus if something strange happens in the yard – like visitors when you don't normally have any. In fact, geese were used to guard nuclear missile silos during the Cold War. The problem with geese though is they defecate all over the place and it's a mess. There is another alternative.

We have several Guinea fowl mixed in with our flock of chickens. They do not have the same messy problem that geese do. The Guineas (or "Gins" as we call them) also raise a ruckus when anything out of the ordinary occurs on our property. This would include cars other than ours pulling in the drive, coyotes or stray dogs in the area and so on. They roam free on the property, and when they are in an area that our outdoor dogs cannot see and raise a ruckus, our dogs go running to investigate. They lay eggs that are fine to eat, they taste like pheasant, and they can fly away from danger. Pretty good system.

Have a safe place to go in your home if trouble occurs. The master bedroom is the obvious choice but you'll have to be able to get the kids in there in an emergency. If not, then you will need to ensure your children stay put in their bedrooms so they don't get in the way of any middle of the night confrontation. I suggest you develop two code words for the kids – one that means "run into Mommy and Daddy's room" and another that means "hide where you are". Make a game of it (no need to scare the little darlings by telling them what it's really for). Perhaps "Bullwinkle!" means run into the master bedroom. Once you teach the kids you must then test them periodically – at all times of the day and night. Reward the winners – heck, reward them all! Keep it fun.

Ideally, you would have a way to secure the sleeping quarters from the rest of the house – a sturdy door, a decorative grill or something similar. Massad Ayoob ("The Truth About Self-Protection") and Jeff Cooper ("To Ride, Shoot Straight, and Speak the Truth") have written on this subject and I defer to them for further advice.

When you go out of town, have a neighbor pick up your newspapers and mail and mow your yard. You could also have the post office temporarily stop delivery if you wanted. As long as we are talking about neighbors – why not try and establish a neighborhood watch? This is a great way to get the community working together before an emergency and it could pay off in the long run.

If you live in a place where it would not be out of place or ostentatious, install a gate at the top of your driveway and use it all of the time. This way, when you go away for a week, no one will notice anything different.

Evacuation or *Bugging Out*

I said earlier that an emergency could arise that would force you and your family to rapidly evacuate your home. Yes, as mentioned above, we all want to stay home with our mountains of survival supplies and network of friends and neighbors. Staying put is almost always the first and best idea. Your government recommends it and so do I. But because we can imagine the unimaginable, we must have a plan for dealing with a situation that would force us from our home and out into chaos. This could be a chemical spill, a raging forest fire, a tidal wave or any of a number of other imminent tragedies.

Bugging out requires one have a plan, the means, and some grab-and-go gear.

The Plan

Let's discuss the plan first. You must have one. First realize you cannot pack a rucksack full of goodies and go live in the woods indefinitely like some modern day Jeremiah Johnson. No, you cannot.

Most folks new to the idea of preparedness put together some kind of survival kit and fantasize about avoiding danger by running to the nearest patch of national forest or other wilderness and "living off the land" like some kind of mountain man. But here's a news flash: the mountain men did not live without support. Most holed up with Indian tribes (civilized society) or wandered into settlements for the winter. They all had to resupply themselves regularly with gun powder, lead balls, salt, and so on. The lone mountain man is pretty much of a myth – most worked with parties of other trappers.

Wild game will quickly become scarce in any kind of full scale crisis. For one thing, there are now a lot more people (potential hunters) occupying the same amount of space over which the Indians and mountain men roamed two hundred years ago. You cannot carry enough food to sustain yourself indefinitely - you need a better plan than that if your family is to survive.

I have had bug out plans originating from several different places (I moved around a lot in my earlier days) and terminating in various locales. I know and have known several people that have workable bug out plans. Based on that, I give you what follows.

The Plan involves:
Start Point
Trigger
Destination
Route
Travel Mode
Supplies

I employ PACE (Primary, Alternate, Contingency, Emergency – multiple options) for almost everything I do. You will do this when you develop The Plan for you and your family.

Start Point

Your primary start point is your home – that's where you spend most of your time and that is where most of your stuff is. Your alternate start point would probably be work or school. Other start points could be wherever you happen to find yourself. If you are planning a three week vacation you may wish to modify your basic plan to suit.

Trigger

You need to decide now what will trigger your evacuation. Do your own threat analysis. Maybe it's a big earthquake, or the Yellowstone Caldera, or nuclear war, or imminent hurricane landfall in your area, or....it's personal. But sit down now and decide what your triggers will be. *What if* them to death. And then, if your trigger trips – GO! Don't think about it - you should have already done all the wargaming you required. When the event is happening is not the time to THINK, it's not the time to DISCUSS, it is not the time to try to GAIN CONSENSUS – it is the time to ACT. Get moving.

Destination

This is the key part of the whole plan. If you don't
have a destination you don't have a plan. Your
destination must be viable – it must support/sustain
you and yours. Selecting the center of the national
forest as your destination will not work. No, it won't.
Not if the only thing there is rocks and trees. You are
not Robinson Crusoe. You are not a mountain man
and even they had support networks.

Your primary destination should be an area that is
outside of the threat danger zone. It should be clear
of the problems that made you flee in the first place.
I suggest you find one at least 150 miles away. This
should get you clear of whatever is immediately
threatening your home. Perhaps you have a relative
living in the next state; maybe an old college buddy
has a place three hours away. You could work out
a deal with them ahead of time that if something
happens at their place they are welcome at yours and
vice versa. You may want to store some supplies at
their place. If they don't have room, consider caching
some there. Or rent a storage unit in their town.

One of my destinations is based on the Yellowstone
Caldera blowing. If it does, we will be moving within
an hour to a location outside of the projected ash fall.
This location is a friend's home. He knows we plan on
coming. Our home is one of his destinations in the
event of problems in his locale. *Quid pro quo.* The key
point here is that both parties need to discuss this
aspect of The Plan and know what they are getting
in for. Your alternate destination needs to be in a
different geographical area. If something happens to
make your primary destination not so nice, you need

to be able to go somewhere else. You need to do all the coordination for this location just like for the primary one. And so on for contingency and emergency destinations.

Another idea, and one which many survivalists choose, is to buy some rural property for a retreat location. You would want it to have water and a means to protect yourself from the elements. You would want to pre-position supplies there as you may end up walking into the place when all is said and done.

Some folks get together with likeminded friends and purchase a piece of property. This can work but it can also end up being a disaster. I suggest you tread carefully. Better to have five acres all your own than to get into a squabble a few years from now concerning your group retreat property.

I said you cannot plan on bugging out to the center of the national forest. Let me caveat that – you cannot plan on it if you have not made any prior preparations. I know of a group that has a bug out location in a mountain town. They own a house there that is stocked with needed supplies and they use it as a vacation cabin. They have also ridden horses into the back country behind their house and cached a robust "spike camp". This is basically tarps and water and food and so on to build a small shanty village in the out back. This is their emergency fallback position.

The best bug out destinations are centered around people. Humans. That you need to talk to. Before hand. You need to develop relationships. This takes effort. This takes time. The vast majority of you are not welcome at Casa Joe during Interesting Times. Nothing personal – we just don't have that kind of relationship. If you plan on fleeing to Aunt Matilda's house – make sure Auntie knows what to expect and agrees. If not – you don't have a plan – you have a wish.

Route

Your route is based on the location of your *Start Point*, the conditions surrounding your *Trigger*, and your *Destination*. Lots of variables, I know. Your primary route should probably be based on the assumption that you are going to get a head start on the masses of fleeing sheep. You will get a head start because you have The Plan and you have your nose to the wind. You will likely (initially) use interstate highways. This is fine for a while.

First, get a current atlas. Yes, the Internet has many useful tools and you *could* print out maps from on line. But an atlas keeps it all together and will cover more areas than you think you need – but might end up needing. Go ahead and spend some time pouring over it. Get very comfortable with your set of maps.

Your alternate route will probably avoid these sheeple magnets and use lesser traveled roads. It will avoid large concentrations of humans. It may avoid military bases – it depends on your envisioned Trigger. I like military bases for most things – but I can legally gain access.

You will have several routes (PACE). Along each one, determine where all of your potential choke points are. Are there bridges, areas subject to traffic jams such as cities, toll booths, and so on? If so, mark them and determine ways around them so that if you need a new route, you will have already planned for it. Are there places along this route where you could stop for fuel (don't count on it in an emergency) or perhaps to pull off the road and rest? If so, mark them. Identify hospitals along your route and anything else you think you could possibly need in time of emergency.

You should have *decision points* along each route where you decided to continue as you are, or switch to an alternative route. Say the New Madrid fault line lets go and you plan to travel along *Route A*. If a bridge is knocked out at what point (on the map and on the ground) will you decide to switch routes? See the section on convoys to read a bit about scouting out decision points enroute.

You need to spend some time on route selection. When you think you know your routes – drive them. Make notes. If the route is viable then designate it Primary or Alternate or..... Then whip out your handy atlas and mark your routes on the map(s). Use different colored highlighters for different routes – this way, if you are injured, someone else can still carry you along your route. Mark any potential hazards or decision points – then decide how you will address them if needed.

You want to plan all of this out now while you are not under stress, while you are well rested and uninjured. You may not be thinking as clearly when it is actually time to evacuate. Plan now.

Travel Mode

Your primary *Travel Mode* will be your "Bug out Vehicle" (BOV). For most of us this is not the purpose-built Uber Vehicle but our daily driver. It does need to be viable in light of the aforementioned aspects of your plan. Deciding to use your Harley to get from Arizona to Maine in February is probably not a good idea. But hey – the point is to think it out – for *yourself.* If you plan on getting to Aunt Matilda's house you better have a way to get there. That rust bucket that can't make it across town will probably not do. You can read more about BOVs later in this book.

Alternate means may be another vehicle, or your neighbor's truck, or a train (you are smart and left *early*) or anything other than your primary vehicle. Other modes could be horse, motorcycle (yeah, I know), or what have you. Your Emergency means will likely be your feet. Your travel mode may affect your routes and location – it all ties together. I was traveling internationally once a long time ago and my personal bug out (get home) plan involved several modes of transportation for each contingency. Perhaps I would drive to the airport and fly home (primary). Perhaps I would take the train to another country, taxi to the airport and fly home (alternate). Or maybe I would book passage on an ocean going vessel with the ample cash I used to carry (it wasn't mine – it was yours. And I gave it back.) Or maybe I would have to take the long walk to the other side of the continent and hook up with some "friends". The point here is that each plan (PACE) must stand alone and not depend on any other plan.

Supplies

Based on what is happening, where you are going, and how you are getting there, you need to decide what you will take with you. If you are going to Aunt Matilda's you may want to ask her what to bring. One of my *Destination* dudes told me not to worry about guns or ammo or clothes or medical gear – "just bring food". Another one told me to bring my goats and chickens! I can carry a lot in my primary bug out vehicle. I cannot carry very much on my back. But I have decided what I will carry with each. You need to plan what you will do if you have to say, abandon your BOVs and hoof it. This is where BOBs come in – can you access yours quickly?

Which brings us to load plans. After you practice and decide how you are packing and where stuff goes - draw a chart - this will greatly speed up the process of getting out of Dodge. Make sure you don't bury the jack underneath fifty gallons of water cans...

Bug Out Vehicles (BOVs)

So you know where you are going and what route you will take to get there. Now you have to think about transportation. Your first option will most likely be by car, SUV, or truck. We call these conveyances BOVs.

You will want a BOV that is mechanically sound and capable of carrying you and your supplies to your retreat location. If you are like most folks, you will have to make do with what you have. If you are in the market for a new vehicle though, you may want to consider some options.

You may want to consider four wheel drive although this is not mandatory by any means. Four wheel drive in and of itself is not enough though. You need to have adequate tires and have some basic skills at driving off road. One way to gain these skills is to join an off-road club. There is probably one in your area.

If you plan on driving off road you will need some specialized tools. High lift jacks, winches, come-alongs, tow straps, shovels, and the like can come in very handy if you get stuck. Again, join an off-road club and you will learn all of this. If you do not join a club, you will have to find some way to practice using your equipment to become unstuck. The time to figure out how to use your gear is not on some dark and rainy night when you are trying to get away from nuclear fallout.

If you must evacuate, you will undoubtedly have to flee your home in the middle of the night, when all gas stations are closed and your fuel gauge is reading a quarter full. Bad news. You should keep your BOV topped off with gasoline and other fluids at all times and have on hand a store of gas adequate enough to get you to your retreat. Perhaps a basket rack could be used to haul the extra gas containers. You will find more information on storing gas in **Light Heat and Fuel.**

The more work you personally do now on your vehicle, the better off you will be when you cannot get a mechanic. If you cannot already do basic repairs – learn! Buy a Chilton's manual, take a class, enlist a buddy – but get your hands dirty and start working on your own vehicles. You can do it. When you work on your vehicle, you will need tools. Buy them. Then you will have them *and* you know how to use them. Bonus.

A list of suggested items to keep in your BOV is located at Appendix F.

You will want enough cargo area. Pickup trucks with a camper shell are great as long as all of the people have a seat. Suburbans and other large SUVs will work also. Whatever you do, please ensure you secure your cargo. Tie it down, bolt it down, or strap it down. You don't want your spare tire or tool box to become a missile headed for the back of your head if you come to a screeching stop.

Camouflage looks cool but it will do the opposite of helping you blend in – it will make you stick out like a sore thumb! You do not want to attract attention to yourself while bugging out. Just make sure your BOV is painted some neutral color. Green, gray, tan, and brown are all good choices.

So, you have your BOV and all is well. At 2 o'clock one morning a fireman pounds on your door and says you have 15 minutes to clear the area as a forest fire is coming up the valley. What do you pack?

A wise survivalist has already thought of this and practiced loading the vehicle. She/he has lists made and knows what goes where. One way to do this is to buy a bunch of Rubbermaid-type containers and play around with fitting them into your cargo space in the most efficient manner. Do this with empty containers. Once you have determined how to totally cube out your space you can then number each bin with a large permanent magic marker and draw a diagram showing what box goes where.
Take your numbered, empty boxes and fill them with

your bug out supplies. Now all you have to do is store your full bins in the garage and periodically have drills where, using your diagram, you load up the vehicle – this will help you to remember and develop little tricks that increase your efficiency.

You may have some items that you cannot afford or don't want to keep stored in bins all of the time. Perhaps it is jewelry, or important papers or the shotgun you keep above the mantel. That's okay – just have a separate list of those items attached to the bins so you can just grab what you need and check it off as you do.

Convoys

If we ever have to use our BOVs for real we will wish, we will *hope* that we have some friends along. Friends with their own BOVs. Let's face it, when the balloon goes up, Murphy shows up. Having spares and buddies is always a good thing when Murphy is lurking in the shadows.

If we ever have to use our BOVs for real – we will want to convoy. I use the word as a verb and a noun. More than one vehicle equals a convoy. It may consist of you driving the BOV while the spouse drives the "daily driver"; it could include friends or team mates - the bottom line is you are traveling together in multiple vehicles from Point A to Point B.

Convoying allows you to carry more stuff, provide for better security, respond to Murphy better, and so on. But, like everything else – you have to think it out ahead of time (we call this planning) and then you have to rehearse. Merely reading about it in an excellent book will not a Convoy Leader make.

The Routes

Everyone in the convoy needs to know where they are headed. We discussed route planning above – it's the same for convoys except that now you factor in more than one vehicle traveling in your party. You will need one map set per vehicle.

The Vehicles

Sure, you'd like to have uparmored HumVees and mine-resistant vehicles but you are stuck with SUVs, pickups and Mom's Corolla. Deal with it. Decide now who is going and what they will drive. Based on what you have, you can determine your movement formations and load plans.

If you had 5 vehicles in your convoy you could have a formation something like: *Scout car* ½ to one mile out front followed the main body consisting of a *Lead vehicle, Front Security, Precious Cargo vehicle* (people or stuff), and *Rear Security.*

You may want a scout vehicle out front. The Corolla would work well here –it's inconspicuous and can drive up to a mile ahead of the convoy proper and report on conditions, warn of road blocks and so on. This vehicle should be "clean" – no heavy artillery. Mom and Pop and a couple bags would be great. We'll get to communications later.

You will want in the convoy proper to have lead and rear security. These are vehicles with firepower (and the best trained operators you have) on board. These are the guys that will respond to problems.

SOPs

You will need SOPs (standard operating procedures) for responding to all kinds of problems: flat tire or mechanical break down, road block, comfort stop, gasoline stop, overnight stop, hostile action, dealing with authorities, light traffic, heavy traffic, and so on and so on. *You* have to decide what you need to plan for. Then sit down and think it out. Come up with a couple different response options and go practice them. Decide on the ones you like as a group and make them your SOPs.

Not every situation will require you to put rounds down range but every situation will require you to ensure 360 degree security. Don't just pull off the side of the road and let everyone gaggle together in a clump... Keep the vehicles spread out but close enough together to control the convoy and keep eyes open all around. You may want to move away from the vehicles – you may not. Think about it now.

You will need a bump plan. Actually, you will need several. They should be written down. If Mike's blue Suburban becomes inoperable, where are the occupants going to ride? What stuff is getting switched over to other vehicles? What stuff is getting dumped out of those vehicles to make room. Decide now – 2:30 a.m. in the rain with bad guys shooting at you from across the highway is no time to have a pow-wow.

Duties
Every vehicle has a driver. The driver's duty is to drive. Period. Every vehicle should have at least one other person. We call this person the TC (Troop Commander) but it doesn't matter. The TC is in

charge of the vehicle and makes the larger decisions. The driver drives and makes immediate decisions (swerve left now!). If there are only two people, the TC reads the map, directs the driver, works the radio and pulls security (looks around and is prepared to respond). It is better if there are more people in the vehicle. It is best if all the TC has to do is read the map and stay situationaly aware and someone else can work the radio. In this case, the TC would be in the front passenger seat and the radio operator can be behind the driver. Everyone should have a piece of the pie around their vehicle to watch while moving and while stopped.

"Unity of Command" is a military principle. "There can be only ONE!" is the battle cry from a cool movie. The point remains. You need one person in charge of the convoy. Pick your leader now. Decisions will have to be made. Some will have to be made and followed immediately – without debate and discussion. If you want to live. Choose wisely.

Communications

Have multiple redundant communications between all vehicles. CBs, FRS, 2-meter, cell phones. Have scanners and radar detectors. Have brevity codes so instead of saying, "HEY, there are dudes with rifles shooting at us from over there, just left of the blue sign" you could shorten that to "Contact LEFT – 10 o'clock". Instead of "we need to stop for gas" you could just say "chocolate milk". Have a code word to switch frequencies.

For routine information you will attract less attention if you use innocuous phrases (like "chocolate milk") rather than if you sound like a military convoy on the

FRS.

Devise signals to use when there are no communications working – flashing lights, hand signals, and the like. Be imaginative but keep it simple.

Gear

Everybody likes gear talk. Every vehicle should be in good repair – if you plan to bug out in it, keep it in good shape. Every vehicle should have basic vehicle stuff – working spare, jack, fluids and so on. Maps, commo and first aid in each BOV. Food and drink. Never separate a person from their BoB – their BoB rides with them no matter what. Never leave a BoB behind to make room for something else.

You should have some serious recovery gear in the convoy – somewhere in the middle or towards the rear. Winches, tow straps, chains, shackles, saws, bolt cutters, come-alongs, crow bars and so on. You should know how to use this stuff.

Consider carrying spare fuel. Decide where you want to carry it. I like carrying mine in roof racks or in a specially designed rack on the back of the vehicle – this saves fumes from leaks affecting occupants. It also makes it more vulnerable to perforation by any of a variety of means.

Once all this is decided, come up with load plans for each vehicle. What goes where in each vehicle? If you are really good standard things (like first aid) will be in the same place in each BOV. Draw a diagram for each BOV showing this and practice loading it to standard.

If you stop overnight, only remove the minimum gear necessary - you may have to leave in a hurry. Keep everything packed up that you are not using. Never separate a person from their BoB. (It bore repeating).

Rehearsals

Practice everything from loading your BOVs, to linkups, to actual movement, to SOPs and so on. After each practice conduct an AAR (after action review) and discuss what you did, what went right, what went wrong, and so on. Ensure everyone participates.

Go back and relook your plans and operations. Tweak them and rehearse again. When you have to bug out for real you don't want the journey to be your first rodeo.

Just as I said earlier that your primary plan should be to stay put, when you bug out, your primary means would probably be by BOV. But Murphy always brings buddies when he shows up. You may load your BOV and take off and then half way to your destination, suffer a catastrophic failure with the vehicle. What do you do now? Do you exit the vehicle, curl up in that fetal position on the side of the road and suck your thumb, muttering "oh dear me"? Nope. You grab your BOBs (one for each fit evacuee) and continue to march. We are not quitters – we are Survivors!

Bug Out Bag

The federal government has said repeatedly that it may take up to 72 hours for any kind of state or federal aid to reach you in such a circumstance. Many hurricane Katrina survivors fled their homes and were on their own for about three days and the media reported the government wasn't doing enough, fast enough. If everyone had assembled "72 hour kits" such as FEMA and the Red Cross had been recommending for years they would have had much less of a hard time.

Since we are survivalists, we realize that problems can come in multiples. That chemical cloud drifting over your neighborhood and forcing you to evacuate could be followed hours later by a nuclear strike on the nation. A pandemic could be ravaging the land and for whatever reason, a group much larger and better armed than you could decide they want your property. Flee or die – we are survivalists so the choice is obvious. You may not be able to ever come home again. There may be no FEMA to take care of you. It could be the end of the world as we know it (TEOTWAWKI).

Since we are survivalists, we like to be a little bit better prepared than the masses and so we have bug out bags or "BOBs". A BOB is a 72 hour kit on steroids and includes a plan.

Being the wise survivalist, you placed your BOBs in quickly accessible locations so that you can grab them and go. Remember I said a BOB is a 72-hour kit on steroids. Think of it as what a backpacker carries on a long hike – but with some extras for contingencies.

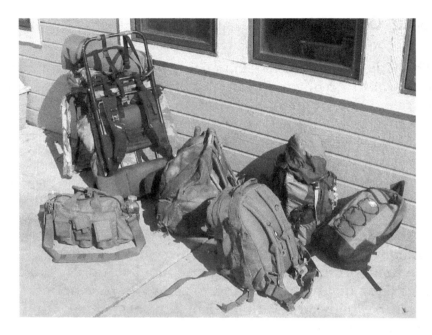

Everyone should have their own BOB. If your child can carry a backpack full of books he/she can carry an individual BOB. This is in case people get separated. Smaller children should at least carry the survival supplies detailed later on in this book. Almost any kind of backpack will do as long as it can hold what you want to carry. What you carry depends on where you are, where you are going, time of year, your physical condition, and the anticipated social environment through which you will travel.

At a minimum, your BOB should contain provisions for the following areas: Water, food, navigation, first aid, shelter, and fire. Remember when I said you cannot live out of your BOB indefinitely? Well that was true. Your BOB is just to assist you in getting to your alternate location.

My family's BOBs have a separate bag of clothing attached to each one. We call this a *Naked Bag*. This is in case we must grab-n-go in the middle of the night when we are wearing pajamas. Each contains underwear, socks, t-shirt, long sleeved shirt, and long pants all tightly rolled up and tied with a bandanna. The clothing is earth toned but not camouflaged. Each bag also contains a pair of boots. In winter, we drape a coat over each BOB as well.

For clothing you will want earth-toned, tough, outdoor type clothes. You can spend hundreds of dollars at a sporting goods store or you can spend only a few shopping at a thrift store. Just remember this: when the balloon goes up no one will be critiquing your fashion sense or lack thereof. You don't want camouflage because in many (and perhaps *most*) instances, you will stick out more wearing BDUs than otherwise dressed. Picture the film clips you have seen of hurricane survivors. Remember the pictures of New York City on 9-11? A whole family looking like militia members will draw unwanted attention.

Our *Naked Bags* are just attached with a snap link so we can grab the entire (unwieldy) package if we must flee scantily clad into the night. But the extra bag can also be quickly jettisoned if we start out adequately clothed.

For water you will want to carry some in your BOB and have a means to collect and purify more. Water is heavy at about eight pounds per gallon. If you are walking with a rucksack you will need at least a gallon a day and probably more. Trying to carry this much will quickly become a self-defeating proposition. It is never a bad idea to pre-select likely water sources along your bug out route(s). You could even cache water along the way. Just buy a case of bottled water and bury it - it will be there when you need it.

You will need food to fuel your trek. I suggest items that can be consumed on the go with limited fuss. Power Bars, EAS bars and other food bars are good. So are jerky, peanuts, crackers and my favorite – peanut butter! Do not worry about "nutritionally complete meals" or vitamin packs – this is a short term proposition. Strap on your BOB and get to your destination. You can eat wholesome food later – what you need now is *Go Food*.

You will want maps of the area and a compass. Make sure you know how to use both. You will also want a first aid kit and possibly tampons and pads for any women. Remember, your goal with your BOB is to get to your destination so focus on mobility items – pain killers, ACE bandages, tape, and so on.

Your primary shelter will be your clothing – make sure it is up to the task. Good walking shoes or boots, rain gear, gloves, hats and so on. We carry a sweater, knit hat and gloves in our BOBs year round. You may also want to add a tarp or poncho to fashion a shelter at night to sleep in. You may even get a small backpacker's tent. You will need something to get out of the weather, catch a short nap and get back on the trail. Remember, you are not going to use your BOB to attempt to live indefinitely in the woods. This is why you have The Plan. This is how you will keep the weight manageable.

You will also want the means to start fire when it is appropriate to do so. Now, having the gear is only part of the equation – you need to have skills as well. These are primarily those camping skills you read about earlier and you can practice them in the back yard if you must.

The types of gear detailed so far are basic components of any survival kit. A BOB *is* a survival kit, albeit a large one - but it is also more.

In addition to the above, you may also wish to include other items. You might have copies of important papers and records such as marriage and birth certificates, inventories of household goods, and so on. Addresses and phone numbers of contacts and family could come in handy. A lot of this could be easily transported via a thumb drive but I like the permanence of paper (adequately waterproofed in a Ziploc bag or two.) To get back into the neighborhood you evacuated, you may need proof of address. A driver's license may suffice but it's tough to keep one in a BOB. You could also use a recent electric bill.

In times of crisis, cash is king. You may want to have some spare cash in smaller denominations – no one will want to make change for you. Some folks I know carry silver and gold to barter with. If you do this, make sure you have it in small enough pieces – tenth ounce gold coins, necklaces, rings, etc. Again, no one is going to give you change for a one ounce gold Krugerrand when you want to buy gas.

Spare glasses and any prescription or daily medications are good things to include. I also carry an empty contact lens case and solution in case my evacuation occurs while I'm wearing my lenses. If you cannot keep a bottle of your daily medications in your BOB at all times – put a large, colorful pull off tag on the BOB that says "MEDS" – that will remind you to run upstairs and grab the bottle from the medicine cabinet before you take off.

Some people carry firearms and ammunition in or with their BOB. Think carefully here. In many situations a gun might be very useful and comforting. In others, it may get you in trouble. My advice here is, *be discreet.*

I keep a small Bible in my BOB because it is an instruction manual for life and I always want one near me. That's just me. Some folks keep a survival manual packed; others, a first aid manual. Hear me on this – you need to *know* basic survival and first aid skills. When you need them, there will be no time to read up on them. The test we are preparing for will be given with no notice. So, carry a first aid book if you must – but please start practicing so that it quickly becomes superfluous.

We live in an area with four seasons and so we have winter and summer BOBs. Well actually, we have a "winter module" that we add to the BoBs when the weather threatens to change. Ours consists of long underwear, a sleeping bag and sleeping pad for each person. Additionally, I carry for the family a tent and a backpacker stove and fuel bottle to quickly prepare warming fluids. When our youngest was too small to carry her own sleeping bag our plan was to slip her into one of ours with us. We never practiced this though and now she is strong enough to carry her own.

You should keep your BOB packed and ready to go at all times. Some keep their BOBs in a closet near the front door, others in the garage, still others in a basement and so on. The key is to have it available at moment's notice. Some folks even keep one at home and one in their commuter vehicle. They call the latter a "get me home bag".

The Test

One Saturday morning several years ago, I asked my wife if she was ready for a pop quiz. I wouldn't say she was overly motivated, but she agreed. I gave her the following scenario: "I am away on a business trip. Something has just happened that is forcing you to immediately flee the house with kids – possibly never to return."

At this point, most people would begin asking a lot of questions such as "What happened?" "What time of year is it?" and so on, but my wife had been through many *"what if?"* scenario discussions and understood my intent.

I started a stop watch and said, "Time starts now and ends when you back the vehicle up." I envisioned her running around the house, grabbing a case of MREs (Meals Ready to Eat –military food that replaced C-rations about 25 years ago) here, a couple jugs of water there, first aid supplies, bedding and so on. In short, I pictured chaos. I planned on watching her pack the vehicle in an unorganized manner and then going over what she selected and seeing if she might have made different choices with the benefit of hindsight.

Instead, my wife called our children downstairs to where she was standing when I popped the quiz, opened the closet and handed each their individual BOBs, shouldered hers, grabbed her keys, looked me in the eye and said, "Do you really want me to back the car up, because we are outta here." Total elapsed time – 20 seconds.

I was floored. "Is that all you are taking?" I asked.

"Yep. You said we had to leave immediately. That's why we have these BOBs, isn't it?" She had me there. She won and I learned something.

You need to use your BOBs. Take yours camping. Take it for walks. I am saddened when I see a BOB full of brand new stuff knowing the owner has never tested it to see if it really works and if it suits *their* needs. Some folks pack BOBs that weigh 80 pounds and "know they can carry it" because they put in on in their living room once." Yeah, right. Take that puppy out for a real walk.

At least twice a year in the summer and winter my family gets together with others for BOB campouts. We pick a remote spot and hike and camp just out of our BOBs to make sure everything is up to par. We have been doing this for years and we still learn something every time.

We bring extras of everything which we leave in the vehicles *just in case.* We consider an individual to have "failed" the exercise if they must go back to the car but we are not going to let anyone get hurt or in trouble for lack of gear. Either way, it's always a learning experience.

We invited a young man, new to survivalism, on one such winter event and thought we had explained the concept fairly well. We parked the vehicles, shouldered our BOBs and hiked a good ways into the woods. Night came quickly and with it snow and sleet. We all quickly rigged shelters from the gear in our packs and then built a large group fire with rock reflector to stay warm. After that was accomplished we all dug into our BoBs for supper. My family heated up Ramen noodles in canteen cups and added foil packets of tuna. Another guy broke out Coast Guard survival rations and a third family opened up some MREs. We were all happily munching away, all of us were also heating up water to make coffee, tea, hot cocoa and so on, and we were feeling pretty good about ourselves. Our new friend rummaged in his BOB and pulled out two steaks wrapped in foil which he plopped into the coals! We ribbed him unmercifully about keeping his BOB "packed 24/7" with steaks in it.

One final note: replace what you use as soon as possible. I learned this lesson the hard way. My family had gone to visit my mother law for the week one summer and on Saturday morning I found myself sitting in front of the computer, surfing the 'net. I suddenly had the idea to give myself a no notice bug out test. It was a Saturday morning; I had nowhere to be and nothing to do until Monday. I was wearing a pair of running shorts, socks and running shoes – that's it. I put a shirt on for propriety's sake, grabbed some dog food, water, bowl, a leash and a cable tie out for my Rhodesian Ridgeback; shouldered my BOB and drove off with my dog to the nearest patch of national forest about two hours away.

This was deep in the Appalachian Mountains and my plan was to park where I usually did when I hunted, change into my "BOB clothes" (which at the time were BDUs) and hike over the ridgeline to the remote valley beyond. I planned to practice some skills, spend the night and return home the next day. I got out of the truck, started changing and realized much, much too late, that I had taken the boots off my BOB the week prior so that I could wear them for some purpose and had failed to replace them. I did hike to the top of that mountain ridge but it was no fun carrying a heavy rucksack up a mountain strewn with rocks and deadfall wearing only running shoes on my feet. I decided not to hike down into that valley – I was risking twisting an ankle and did not want to turn this into a real survival situation. Lesson learned – replace what you use! It helps to place a note on the BOB reminding yourself.

You will find a list of contents of an adult and a child's BOB at Appendix G.

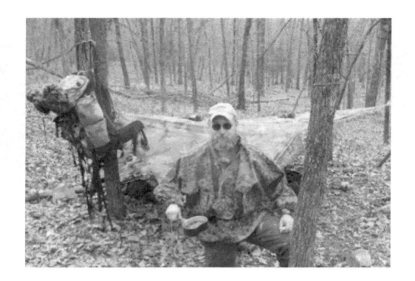

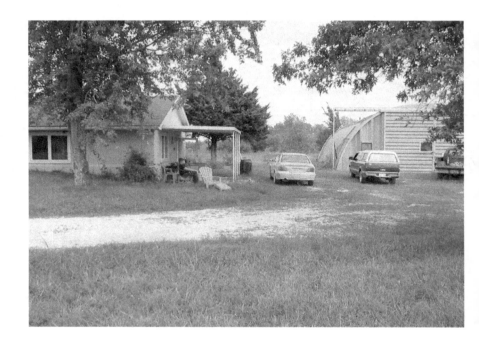

TAKING IT TO THE NEXT LEVEL

Water

As a survivalist family, you need to have a plan to provide for your own water. I teach my wilderness survival students *The Rule of Threes* as a way to prioritize survival needs: You can live three minutes without air, three hours without shelter, three days without water and three weeks without food. Air refers not only to breathing but also includes blood (which carries oxygen). Shelter covers things like hypo- and hyperthermia. So we come to water. You will die if you go more than a couple days without it. Therefore, it's pretty important, despite the fact that we rarely think of it. To survive you would need a quart or two a day – that's just to sit there. A rule of thumb bandied about is to store one gallon per person per day. This will provide for your drinking and cooking needs and leave you a little to wash up with. If you want a shock, check your water bill from last month and see how much water you use per person per day. Now obviously, in survival situations you will not use that much water but you will want *at least* a gallon per person per day. With water we are concerned about three major things: acquiring it; purifying it; and storing it.

Acquisition
When your taps stop working you can still get a short term supply of water from your home. The first thing you'd want to do is turn the incoming water off at the

main valve – thus trapping all the water you do have in the pipes. You need to know where this valve is anyway incase you have a burst pipe or something later. Go find it and show the kids – it's usually on the wall closest to the street, usually in the washroom, basement, or other "unfinished" area.

Once you've done that you can start at the top of the house and work your way down opening taps and draining water into suitable containers. Leave the taps open so air can flow in the pipes and allow the lower water out. You also have clean water in the back of every toilet – that is unless you add that blue stuff to the tank. Your major source of household water though will be your hot water tank – they typically hold 35 – 50 gallons of fresh water. You can drain if from the spigot at the bottom. All of this water is tap water and should be just fine.

There are other water sources for you to *tap* into which you would have to purify if you planned on drinking or cooking with it. You may be able to divert rain water from your down spouts into large containers. You could certainly set out containers to catch rain. If the containers are clean and the rain touches nothing else on the way down you really wouldn't have to purify it either. You could stretch out a large tarp lifted up on the ends by boxes or perhaps placed in a low spot and it would act like a giant sink collecting rain. You may have a swimming pool or fish pond. Perhaps there is a stream or pond nearby from which you could haul water.

Some old houses have cisterns into which the roof gutters used to flow. As cities built up many of these were filled in or had the water diverted. If you live in a hundred year old house you may want to investigate whether or not you have such a cistern. I know some folks who hand dug a well at their place – just to have water "if they need it".

Purifying

Most of this outside water will need to be purified. A time tested method is to boil it. If you bring the water to a full rolling boil you will kill the nasties therein. The key here is "full rolling boil". Just to make sure, it's a good idea to boil it for a couple minutes. Boiling sounds simple enough, right? It is, but you have to consider how you will boil it and what container(s) you will use. Will you do it in a saucepan over a Coleman stove or in a stock pot outside on a grate over a fire pit? Whatever method you choose, ensure you have enough fuel for your needs.

You can purify water with water purification tablets and this is a good idea for Bug out Bags and 72 hour kits, but this is not really a good long term option – it would get very expensive, very quickly.

You can also use bleach to purify your water. You want bleach with a 5.25 to 6% concentration of sodium hypochlorite. First filter out as many impurities as possible by running the water through a few towels, or coffee filters or something similar. Then add 16 drops of bleach per gallon, stir it up, and let it sit for thirty minutes. After that time it should have a slight chlorine smell – if it doesn't, add sixteen drops, stir, wait and sniff again. If it still has no chlorine smell you have really bad water – get rid of it and seek water elsewhere!

Yet another way to purify water is to use ceramic filters. You can purchase large countertop models like the Big Berkey or you can get handheld pump types such as Katadyn and Pur from camping stores. These screen out incredibly small organisms and are guaranteed to provide good drinking water. Different filters are rated to purify differing amounts of water. Bigger filters obviously filter more and dirty water lessons the life span of any filter. Best check before buying.

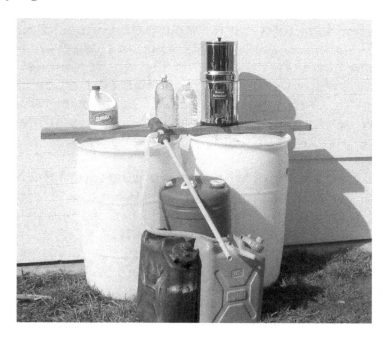

Storage

You will want to have a certain amount of water stored for your family. How much you store is up to you based on your own assessments. It is also based on the amount of space you have available. Water is heavy – in fact it weighs about eight pounds per gallon.

Water will not "go bad". There is no expiration date despite what you may read on bottled water. If you store clean water in a clean container and keep it away from light it will last indefinitely. If your water goes flat from long storage simply pour it back and forth from one (clean!) container to another to aerate it. You will want to keep it away from sunlight or you stand the risk of growing algae in your drinking water.

Some people buy cases of bottled water for their emergency needs. This is a viable but very expensive solution. Tap water is much cheaper.

I used to store water in washed out milk containers. *Do not do this*. First off, they are a pain to clean properly – you have to ensure all of the milk is out as well as all of the soap. Secondly, because they are designed to break down in a landfill, they will start to leak on you eventually. I found this out the hard way after storing several gallons underneath the stairs and behind several cardboard boxes of supplies. Go thou, and do not likewise.

Empty two liter soda bottles are great for storage. We just rinse them out twice with tap water, fill them up and then stick them in dark closets. I had a friend give me several special purpose built racks designed to hold these bottles when transporting them via a hand truck into a store. This allows me to stack racks of six bottles up to about four racks high. I keep a couple of these bottles in each vehicle and they handle freezing well if you only fill them about 2/3 full.

If you want to get even more serious about water storage you can get plastic containers in capacities from five to sixty gallons. You can buy these brand new from a variety of distributors for about one dollar per gallon capacity or you can get them very cheap to free from cola bottling plants. Look them up in your nearest city yellow pages. These bottling plants get the ingredients for soda trucked in in large barrels that they use once and then discard. You will have to clean them out before storing your water in them. I first used Dawn dishwashing detergent and then after thoroughly rinsing them I refilled the barrels and added baking soda and let them sit in the sun for a few days – this did an adequate job. I'm not sure how much longer this resource will be around though as I have noticed the bottling plants are starting to use large Mylar bags for the cola syrup and what not.

If you store your water in barrels you will undoubtedly store it outside. This is fine – just make sure no sunlight hits your barrels. To prevent the formation of algae add eight drops of bleach to each gallon of water (from the tap and already chlorinated). You will also want to double tarp it. Cover the barrels first with black plastic and then with a dark tarp. I typically rotate this water once or twice a year just for peace of mind and to check on algae formation.

You will also want to ensure that your barrels are only 2/3 full if your area gets deep freezes. This will allow for expansion of ice. You will have to have some means of melting the ice for water if you need it in winter. Solar heat comes to mind. So does rolling the barrel into a warmer room.

Sixty gallons of water weighs about 480 pounds. Not the easiest thing to move around. Buy some hand pumps – referred to as "siphon pumps" to extract your water when needed. Failing that, you can use a length of water hose as a siphon – just like siphoning gas but not as gross!

Food

Why do you need food storage? Well stuff happens. There could be a national emergency – maybe a truckers' strike. There could be a local emergency like a deep winter storm. You could have a personal emergency such as the loss of your job and income. In any case, if you have your food needs met, it will allow you to think and plan your next move without the panic that accompanies an empty larder and no immediately clear means of obtaining more food. I had a friend who was unexpectedly laid off from his job. He was already living on the margins but his 4 children did not go hungry during the two months it took him to find another job because he had a pantry full of food.

I for one do not want to picture my children hungry, no food to be found anywhere, and me having to solve that problem. I have taken steps to avoid that by implementing a food storage program – I suggest you do the same. Of course, how much food you store is up to you. You know how to do a threat assessment now – how much food do *you* think you need?

You will want to keep your food "cool, dark, and dry" to maximize the nutritional shelf life. This means the closer you can keep it to 40 degrees the better it will last. Heat, light, and moisture will all negatively impact your food storage. Properly canned food rarely goes bad – it just loses nutritional value over time. You can compensate for that somewhat with a supply of good multi-vitamins.

You also want to keep your food bug and mouse free. We store food such as pasta and flour in large Rubbermaid tote bins and we throw several bay leaves into each container – this supposedly keeps bugs away and it has worked for us in many different environments.

Keep a tidy pantry – don't let food sit around open. Keep an eye on things in there and when needed, get the mouse traps out.

You want to rotate your food stores so that you are continuously eating the oldest food. The golden rule is "Store what you eat and eat what you store." If you go out and purchase a year's worth of "survival food" that you only plan on eating in an emergency, at some point (if no emergency occurs in that time) the food is going to get too old to use. You will then pretty much have to throw it away and buy more. Not very economical.

You can break your food storage down into three main areas – short, medium and long term storage. As I mentioned, it really depends on your personal assessment how much food you decide to store. The federal government advises everyone store at least three weeks of food – two weeks in the home, three days worth in a "72 hour" or "grab and go" kit and three days worth in your vehicle. The Church of Jesus Christ of Latter Day Saints (Mormons) advises their members to have a year's worth of food. If you want to store more than a year's worth of food it gets difficult to rotate and you may want to consider becoming self sufficient in your food production by planting large gardens, raising domestic animals and so on. This is getting into the homesteading realm and is outside the scope of this book.

Short Term Storage

Short term food was discussed earlier in **The Basics** and consists of things you can eat with little or no preparation such as Spaghetti-os, granola bars, tuna fish and so on. Just ensure you have enough on hand at all times to take care of your potential future needs.

Medium Term Storage

Most folks run into problems with medium term food storage – food for a few months. You may have to change your eating habits if you want to rotate your food stores. For example, one friend of mine ate out about three or four times a week. It is tough to rotate through a couple months worth of food when you eat out that much. My family loves fresh vegetables but we realize we need to have canned vegetables in our food storage program so we force ourselves to eat canned goods a few times a week – just to ensure we rotate our supplies. Good medium term storage foods include pasta, beans, rice, canned goods, flour and crackers (good for up to a year if you can control the humidity).

We have a 4 tier storage system. The first consists of canned goods on what I call "Mormon shelves" (I got the idea from an LDS friend). The shelves are set at an angle along the long axis so the cans roll to the bottom. We load new cans on the high side and use the cans from the low side – thus insuring we rotate our supplies.

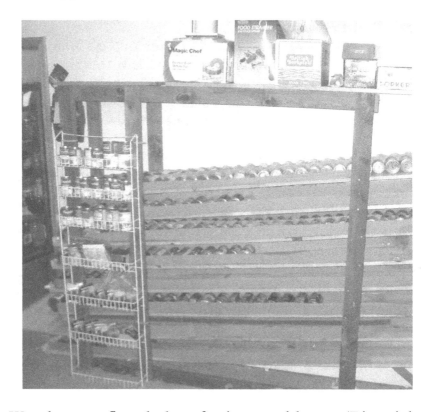

We also use flat shelves for jars and boxes (Bisquick, PopTarts), bins for stuff like flour, sugar, and crackers, and buckets for miscellaneous items such as candy and spices. We also have long term storage consisting of wheat, corn and rice in sealed buckets.

When my family began storing food we sat down and calculated how much of each item we wanted to store based upon our own threat assessments. We then went out and, over time, bought all the food we felt we needed. We now judge our level of storage by how empty the shelves look. We know "what right looks like". When we start getting low on, say, peas - it's easy to see that the peas shelf is missing a few cans. It's not quite that simple because we usually buy in case lots and so when we are "low on peas" we usually buy a case and not just a few, so some end up sitting on the floor. When the flour bin looks low, we buy more flour and so on. We aren't list keepers.

We have similar "comfort levels" for our dog food bags (we stack them up on top of each other) and chicken and horse feed. When they look low - we buy a good bit more.

You can save a good deal of money purchasing food this way. Whereas one family may stop by the store to pick up a couple cans of corn for supper – and pay full price, we are able to wait until there are sales when we purchase several cases. I refuse to shop in stores that limit the number of sale items a customer may purchase – when something goes on sale, I want to buy a lot. Much of the food we eat was purchased on sale. The trick here is to have enough in storage to allow you to take advantage of sales and to only purchase foods you are going to eat.

Long Term Storage
The final category of food is long term storage. This is food that will last a long time and could include wheat, corn, beans, cooking oil, salt, and sugar or

honey. This is basically what the Mormon church recommends. I talk about LDS a lot because they figured out food storage a while ago and provide excellent resources.

Wheat found in Egyptian tombs was sprouted thousands of years later. Wheat is good for survival food storage! But there are some challenges to overcome. The first is how to prepare it. You will need a grinder or mill. There is an entire section below dedicated to these wonderful tools.

You will have to learn how to cook and bake with flour. The way to do this is to, well, DO it! Start baking bread – your family will love you for it. You can also make flat and pan breads on the stove top and hushpuppies, doughnuts and the like in a deep fryer. You can also make cereal (gruel) from wheat but I do not like it.

You want to ease into a whole wheat diet a little at a time – use white flour mixed with your wheat flour at first until your digestive track gets used to it. White flour will store for several years if you keep it cool, dark, dry and bug free.

Putting it up
You can pay a premium and get your corn and wheat pre-packaged in nitrogen sealed buckets or you can save yourself a lot of money and do it yourself. Simply go to the local feed store (if don't live in the country you will get to take a drive!) and buy it by the fifty pound sack. It is so cheap as to be ridiculous.

On the way home, stop by the local Chinamart and purchase white five-gallon buckets and lids in the paint section. You will need about one bucket per thirty pounds of product. Buy some kitchen sized trash bags while you are at it – the inexpensive, unscented, untreated kind.

On the day you want to put up your supplies, go out early and purchase some dry ice. Look around for it – grocery stores have it, ice cream stores sometimes do as well. Bring it home in a cooler. Line each bucket with a trash bag. Wearing gloves, smash up the dry ice with a hammer into fist sized chunks and drop one into each bucket then immediately fill the bucket with grain. Give the bag a half twist and set the lid on top. Do not seal the lid. Very soon fog will start pouring out of the buckets – this is carbon dioxide (CO_2) which is displacing the oxygen (O_2) in your containers. Let them sit there until it stops pouring out.

Since CO_2 is heavier than oxygen as long as you don't disturb the buckets there won't be a lot of oxygen in the bucket when you seal the lid 30 minutes or so later. Simply twist the bag shut and snap the lids on. I then wait an additional hour or so to ensure I don't get and exploding bucket at which point I use duct tape around the lid to completely seal off the bucket.

What you have just done is deny oxygen to any critters living or getting ready to hatch in your wheat. If you fail to do this, when you go to open your bucket months later you could find nothing but powder and dead bugs.

Another way to store grain is to mix it with diatomaceous earth (DE). DE is actually fossilized sea creatures with very sharp microscopic projections.

You cannot see or feel them – DE looks like flour. You simply mix in a couple cups of DE per fifty pounds of product (such as rice) and then place in bucket and seal up. The easiest way to do this is to pour the rice into a large bin and then mix in the DE with your hands per the instructions. When the bugs hatch (oh yes, there are eggs in there) they will have there microscopic exoskeletons damaged by the DE and they will dehydrate and die. You will not be able to see them. DE is fine for human consumption – it won't hurt you at all in the amounts specified.

You can kill the eggs that exist in your food such as flour, wheat, beans and so on by freezing it for three days and then placing it in a bug proof container. This is good to remember if you ever notice an eruption – put your affected food in the deep freeze (or on the back porch if it's the right time of year) and you will take care of the problem. After freezing, just ensure that no oxygen or moisture can reach your product and you will be fine.

Balance and Variety

You will want to provide for a balanced diet. Remember to add a good multi vitamin to your stores. The only way I've found to rotate these is buy a large supply and take one a day. Keep your extra vitamins in the freezer.

You will probably want to provide for some variety. This is not absolutely necessary though – many people on this earth eat basically the same thing every day. Americans consume more sugar per capita than any other nation – to avoid "culture shock" you might want to add some sweets to your stockpile as well.

Here are some ideas for foods that store well in various categories:

Protein - tuna, sardines, smoked oysters, canned ham, chicken, etc; peanut butter, jerky, sausages, Macaroni and cheese/rice and beans/corn and beans – eaten during the same meal.

Vegetables – canned, dehydrated

Fruits – canned, dehydrated, jellies, jams, juice, fruit leathers

Starch – pasta, wheat, flour, Ramen noodles, corn, cornmeal, cake mixes

Drinks – juice boxes, Kool-aid mixes, coffee, tea

Sweets – sugar, chocolate, hard candies, cocoa

Cooking

Now that you have your food storage taken care of – how will you prepare it and clean up afterwards?

Having an extra bottle of propane for the gas grill will take care of most short term emergencies. If you have a charcoal grill you could purchase several bags of charcoal when they go on sale and know that you are taken care of for awhile. By the way, you don't need starter fluid to get charcoal burning. You can light a small fire of sticks surrounded by your briquettes or you could use one of those tube "charcoal starters" into which one places a single sheet of crumpled up newspaper.

Small camp stoves will do in a pinch also. The thing about all three types of stoves (gas, charcoal, camping) is that you need fuel. When you run out of fuel the stove will not work. Well, you could still build small fires in a charcoal grill and use that. So, ensure you have enough fuel stored.

Fuel really should be stored in a shed or other structure separate from your home and garage. You just want to keep it dry and away from other combustibles. If you do have to store it in a garage, make sure you take every possible precaution to avoid fires. You can read more about this in **Light Heat and Fuel**

You may want to build an outdoor fire ring and learn how to cook over a campfire. If your ordnances prohibit doing so now, you could learn at the local national forest or campground. You will want to know how to prepare meals over a fire before it becomes the only way to do so. As you begin to cook more and more over fire you will undoubtedly acquire and grow to love cast iron cookware. If you have children – enroll them in scouts and sign yourself up as an adult leader. You DO have time – it's for the children.

Gear
As you begin to cook more and more over fire you will undoubtedly acquire and grow to love cast iron cookware. We cook on cast iron everyday and when we go camping we take along some of it. I love returning from a campout and using the same cast iron frying pan we used over a campfire recently. We may be cooking up bacon and eggs in the kitchen at home but we can still smell hints of wood smoke on that pan for a few days.

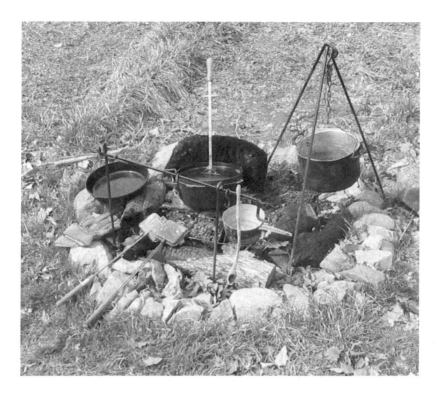

Cast iron is good because it transfers the heat equally and efficiently, it is tough and there are no plastic parts to melt off in or near a campfire. We own several cast iron frying pans of varying sizes and we use them every day. Supposedly, if you use a metal spatula while cooking with cast iron, you will get enough iron in your diet. I dunno – but it sounds good to me!

Dutch ovens

In addition to frying pans, you will want a Dutch over or two. In one of these you can cook stew, bake bread or a cake, roast meat, and in fact – you can even use the inside of the lid as a frying pan. They come in several styles an you will generally want one with legs (to hold it up above the coals and let air flow) and with

125

a rim around the lid (to hold coals on top). I have even seen Boy Scouts stack several Dutch ovens on top of each others in a tower-like affair with coals on top of ever lid and thus cook several things simultaneously. We also have a Dutch oven with no legs and we use it on our stove at home as a deep fryer as well as making awesome pot roasts in it. Details of how to cook with a Dutch oven are beyond the scope of this book but there are many good resources on the Internet - just google "dutch oven cooking".

Pots

Cast iron is wonderful but it is heavy. You don't need to be lifting some monstrous cast iron kettle on and off the fire just to cook up some spaghetti noodles or heat up some green beans. For simple tasks like that a sturdy enamel ware, aluminum, or light stainless steel pot will work wonders. Our aluminum "camp pot" was found in a roadside trash pile. We took it camping the first time and quickly realized it needed a bail (handle) to suspend it over the fire. I fashioned one out of some heavy gauge wire laying about and we have used it that way ever since. Oh sure, I could replace it with a nicer looking one but we have grown used to this one and it's kind of nostalgic.

I have heard some bad things about cooking with aluminum pots – stuff like it can cause Alzheimer's or something. I have no idea if this is true or not but we did get rid of all of our aluminum pots save the large camp pot and we don't use that one every day. You do your own research and make your own decisions here.

Tools

Cast iron gets hot. You will want some heavy duty leather gloves (we keep a dedicated set in our camp box) to use when adjusting your pots and pans over the fire, removing them altogether, and so on. You will also want a "Dutch oven lid lifter" This is a lever type deal that lets you achieve some stand off as you move your Dutch oven around and when you remove the (very hot) lid. The longer your lever, the more you will like it. You will also want a shovel to move coals around and a brush to clean the lid before lifting.

You will want a grill to span the sides of your fire and on which you will set pots and pans for frying and boiling. I use the pull out grills from old ovens. Do not use metal refrigerator grates - they are not up to the task and many contain noxious substances that you don't want in your fire.

There are numerous campfire cooking gadgets out there from coffee pots to pastry makers. My advice to you is to start cooking over fire and determine what works for you. Scouting is a great organization and participating will allow you to see a lot of different techniques and equipment – there's yet another plug!

Seasoning

Well used and properly prepared cast iron works a lot like Teflon pots and pans – without the delicateness that makes such gear unsuitable for campfire cookery. Before you use cast iron you must "season" it. Basically wash it will with something like Dawn dishwashing detergent and then dry it well. Next you will rub cooking oil onto all surfaces – inside and out. Some people use vegetable shortening like Crisco. You

don't need a lot but you do need full coverage.
After cleaning and oiling you need to heat it up. Either
place it in an oven and turn the heat to 350 degrees
(let the pot warm up with the oven) or better yet –
place it in your grill outside or on a campfire. You
"bake" the piece until it stops smoking and then let it
cool on the fire, in the stove, or whatever. This process
sets the oil and makes it into a fairly durable surface.

Easy Clean Up

Okay, you've broken into your food storage, you fired
up the grill and cooked your family a fine meal of oh,
chili or spaghetti. How are you going to clean up? We
can't have dirty dishes around the place.

Since you just read about cast iron, we will begin
there. When you clean your cast iron, you do not use
soap – just scrape it out, wipe it out or let it boil out
and then reapply some oil. You do not need to season
it again unless you use soap on it or scour it too hard
with a scrubbie. The more you use your cast iron – the
nicer it gets.

As far as eating utensils go, you can use paper plates
to eat off of and burn them (fuel?) when done. Another
way is to eat foods that require little or no preparation.
I eat instant oatmeal everyday at work for breakfast. I
simply pour hot water from the coffee maker into the
little envelope of oatmeal and stir it up with a spoon.
When I'm done, I lick off the spoon and toss the empty
package in the trash – no clean up. Foods like this are
fine for short term situations.

If you get into a long term scenario though, you will
want to eat better meals – meals like the spaghetti
mentioned above. Even if you eat off of paper plates,

you will still have pots to clean. You may read more about properly cleaning up in **Hygiene**.

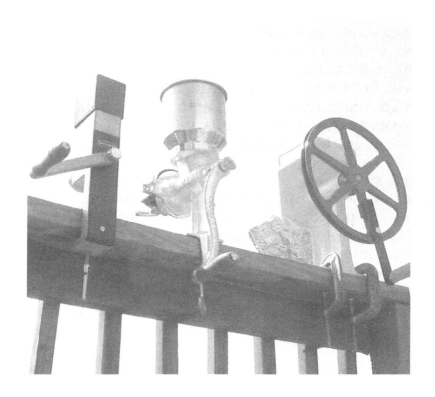

Grinders and Mills

Dried whole grains form the basis for any serious long term food storage program. Dried whole grains can also be used for medium term food storage programs at significant cost savings over more processed foods. Example – a pound and a half of corn meal costs about what? Three bucks? So for a ten spot I could get four and half pounds of corn meal. For that same $10 I can get fifty pounds of dried corn at the feed store. What's the difference between fifty pounds of dried corn and the same amount of corn meal? A grinder and a couple hours of effort.

The example above used corn. We can see similar cost savings with flour and wheat. Around here, 50 pounds of hard red winter wheat costs $12. Wheat, properly stored lasts forever. Flour, due to the milling process can go rancid after a period of time so not only is it more expensive, it is also less durable. The difference between whole wheat grain and flour? A grinder.

Back to Basics

The first wheat grinder (I call them grinders but I think the proper term is mill) we bought was the Back to Basics grain mill. It cost about $60 pre-Y2K and it's not much more expensive now. It is quite small – about the size of a carton of cigarettes. It works fine for grinding wheat into flour. Over the years, I have ground wheat for many a loaf of bread – nothing like home made bread from wheat you ground yourself.

It works "okay" for grinding corn into meal. The steel plates are adjustable – a bit, but corn is oilier than wheat and it gets clogged up at times necessitating taking it apart and brushing off the mechanism with an old toothbrush I keep for just that purpose. When milling corn one must also poke around in the hopper (I use a chopstick) to keep the corn flowing. But again, wheat grinds up just fine with no problems.

Corona

Because of the problems we had grinding corn with the Back to Basics mill we searched about for another, more suitable option until we found the Corona. This is the AK-47 of grain mills – it is tougher than woodpecker lips and being "manufactured from the finest quality cast iron" it weighs about as much as an AK. It is made in Colombia by and for people who know all about grinding corn. It costs less than $40 and grinds corn into perfect meal like nobody's business.

I recently gave a class on grinding, milling and processing various foods and we tried to grind some wheat in our Corona. First pass through – not so good. Very rough texture. Second pass through – it was okay but not great. The Corona is for corn and I guess in a pinch wheat - but really it was designed for corn. And it does a great job with it. I love this mill.

Country Living Grain Mill
I pinched pennies and saved for years until I could finally afford this mill. It is so popular in the more serious preparedness circles that it even has its own acronym – CLGM. We bought ours for around $350. They are now about $400. I also purchased with this mill the "Power Arm" and having tried using it with and without, I would advise you to spend a little extra and get one. I did not buy the chute which guides the flour into the bowl one places beneath the mill when grinding. Instead, I just tape a piece of aluminum foil to the mill and shape it as needed. Ugly but cheap and effective.

The CLGM is better – much better than the Back to Basics mill. It grinds wheat faster, it feels more rugged and it has a groove in the fly wheel that would allow one to hook it up to a belt driven system (driven by an electric motor, a bicycle, a two arm deal – whatever you can imagine and fashion) to make the grinding even easier. Is it over $300 better? I will say this –

I'm glad I bought it but I would not feel slighted if all I could afford was the Back to Basics. They both grind wheat to fine flour. If you have the money – buy one. If you don't – the first one will work for you.

Porkert

And finally we come to a real grinder. This is another "AK-47-tough" piece of equipment and this one is made in the Czech Republic and sold all over the world for grinding meat. Mine cost about $35 and came with a variety of grinding plates and sausage stuffers that hook right on. We bought it for grinding venison into hamburger and have only used it once.

Those familiar with butchering venison will know that each muscle is surrounded by fascia ("silver skin") and let me tell you – that stuff gums up a grinder. I have been told that freezing the meat first and then grinding helps with this but when my wife and I put up a deer we *put up a deer.* Today. We don't have an over abundance of freezer space to use for prepping meat to be ground. So now, when we want venison "hamburger" like for chili or spaghetti or something we take out a package labeled "chunks" and mince it with a big ol' razor sharp butcher knife. When we want beef hamburger we buy it that way.

I suppose we could get beef at the store and grind it up for sausage but honestly, we don't eat a lot of sausage. We don't eat pork as a general rule either so there ya go. My buddy raises cattle though so maybe some day we will be grinding some serious burger. But until then – it sits on a shelf unused in the pantry.

Conclusion

Grinders and mills have a place in any serious survivalist's supplies. Start saving your pennies and get yourself one or two. Do not wait to buy your grain however, until you get a grinder. Get the grain right now. Today. Cresson Kearney shows us how to make a primitive mortar and pestle with a coffee can and a few pieces of rebar in his book Nuclear War Survival Skills. Heck if all you had was the grain you could grind it on your concrete patio or drive way with a brick if you had to.

But you really don't have to, now do you? You could buy a mill instead. When you buy your mill(s) make sure you also buy spare parts. When you need a part you can pretty much be sure UPS won't be delivering if you catch my drift...

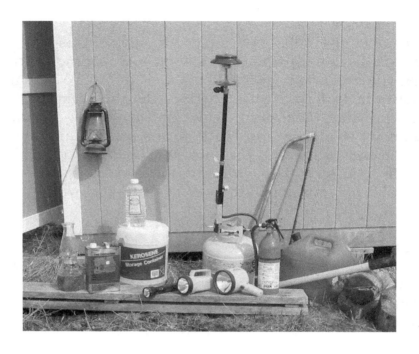

Light Heat and Fuel

In **The Basics** we covered the need for some flashlights and batteries. Every member of your family should have one next to the bed. You should have at least one in every vehicle. Make sure you check your batteries often. Make sure you keep a good supply of extra batteries – they are one of the first things people buy in an emergency. You may wish to consider purchasing rechargeable batteries and a solar recharger – it should save you money in the long run.

Candles are an old standby for lighting. Just make sure you have stable candle holders and keep some extra fire extinguishers around. You can increase the

134

light output of your candles with mirrors or even shiny aluminum foil. We place our candles (in holders) on a piece of aluminum foil and place a mirror behind them. You can also buy or make a candle holder to carry around the house – the kind with a reflective surface behind the candle. You could make one out of a tin can by slicing a large "I" in the side and peeling back the wings.

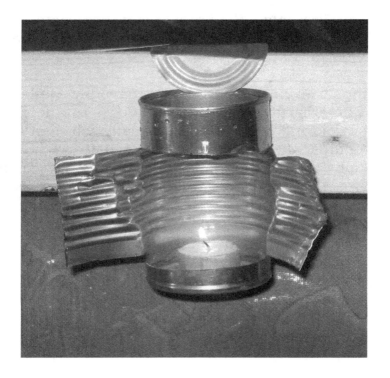

Save your old melted wax to make additional candles or to make fire starters. To do that you would place the pieces of wax into a can onto which you have fashioned a wire handle – coat hangers work well. Suspend this can into a pot of boiling water. When the wax melts, you pour it over dryer lint you have stuffed into cardboard egg cartons and let it cool. You should set your egg carton on a piece of aluminum foil so any leakage does not ruin your table or other work surface. Be careful – melted wax is hot and can injure you!

When you want a fire, simply rip off an "egg" and light the edge. These starters burn very hot for several minutes. Of note: You never want to melt wax directly over a heat source – use a double boiler type method to avoid a fire. Also, the lint works if it consists primarily of natural fibers (cotton, wool) – if you have mostly polyester lint it will not work.

Oil lamps with hurricane globes are readily available at most Chinamarts and through catalogs. You need not buy the colorful "lamp oil" they usually sell right next to the lamps. Just buy K1 kerosene instead – it is essentially the same thing for a lot less money. There are more rugged kerosene lamps – kind of like the old train conductors used to use. I recommend you buy quality here – in my experience the Chinese knock offs don't hold up well to sustained use.

These lamps can put off some smoke and you will definitely smell it if not see it. You can mitigate this by turning the lamp wick down and by ensuring proper ventilation. You should also periodically trim your wick per the directions that come with the lamp. Speaking of wicks – buy a bunch. They are cheap and not that easy to make on your own.

Coleman white gas lanterns works well and provide a lot of heat in a little package. With these you would want to purchase many extra mantels – the net bag that glows when lit. If you buy one of these lanterns it pays to spend a few more bucks and get the plastic case to hold it. This will help prevent broken glass.

Solar power is a whole different and exciting area. You can get lights varying from the little ones that line a walkway to solar powered security lights to whole households run on solar. I do not have solar yet and do not feel qualified to discuss it in detail.

One thing I do know about solar is that with the proper windows, you can heat up your house with just plain old solar gain on a sunny, winter day. If you have windows on the south and west sides of your house you will have not only light but a heat source as well – assuming you have good, air tight, multi-pane windows.

One of the easiest ways to keep warm is to wear more clothes. Sounds simple, huh? We keep our thermostat set at 60 in the winter and just wear layers. There really is no need to heat a house while you are sleeping in most of the country – just pile on more blankets and turn the heat back up upon awakening. Now obviously you don't want a freezing house – that's bad for water pipes but if you have an adequately insulated home, you should be able to turn the thermostat down at night with little fear of burst water pipes.

Wood stoves can be a blessing to a cold home. Just make sure it is properly installed and you keep the chimney clean. Again – buy fire extinguishers and practice fire drills. If you have a wood stove you will need wood. You should have the means to cut and split more. Chainsaws are expensive and must be maintained – but they beat the heck out of a two man cross cut saw! Buy fuel, oil, spark plugs, sharpeners, spare chains, perhaps a spare bar and so on to ensure you have a working saw when you need it. And yes, buy a cross cut saw and sharpening files as well.

We split our own wood with mauls, wedges, sledge hammers and axes. It's good exercise. I suggest you get tools with fiberglass handles and if you have wood tools to purchase a few spare wood handles. You will break some.

You will want to keep your firewood pile away from the home if termites are a problem in your area. You should cover the pile with something to keep the wood dry. Tarps work okay but you have to tie them down (and thus untie them when want your wood) to keep them from blowing away. A wood shed with a roof is a better idea.

Kerosene heaters are very reasonable and can heat a large area. Kerosene stores for a long time with no special treatment. Just make sure you have the heater in a place that it will not get bumped over and did I mention fire extinguishers yet? You will need kerosene of course. Best to figure out how much ahead of time and lay in a supply.

There are little propane heaters on the market also – I have not yet used any but the look like they would be okay for short term needs. As with everything else, you will need fuel.

Survivalists store a lot of fuel – gasoline, propane, white gas, kerosene and so on. As you start stocking up on fuel you need to find a place to store it. Keeping many gallons of flammables in your garage or basement is asking for problems. The best thing to do is keep the fuel in a separate shed 100 feet or more from any other structures. Make sure it is well ventilated and the cans are off the ground. Be nice to your local firefighters and mark the outside the shed correctly.

If you are going to store your gas for several months at a time you will want to treat it with an additive such as Stabil. It is very easy to use - just add a little per the instructions to your gas can, shake and you are done. I only use Stabil on gasoline that I have cached along various bug out routes. For gas storage at home I simply rotate the supply by emptying all of my cans every month into my vehicles and then filling them back up.

Medical

As far as medical concerns go you need to cover four basic areas: information, medicine, supplies, and training.

Information

You should have several in-depth books and or computer print outs covering the various medical subject areas. You *should* read them now but even if don't it would be nice to have the references later if you needed them. Consider texts on nursing, drugs, symptoms, and advanced first aid.

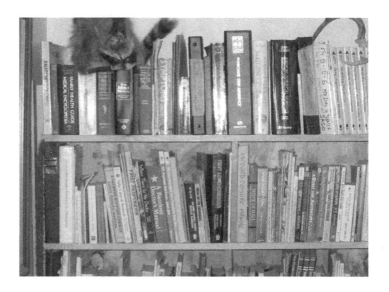

Medicine

By now you already know that you need a supply of everyday medications. You probably want to stock up on "common medicines" like cold medicines, anti-diarrheals, fever and pain medications and so on.

NOTE: I am not a medical professional. You must verify any medical information you get from this book with a medical professional who can take your particular circumstances into account. I am merely reporting what I believe and have used – I take no responsibility for how you use or misuse this information.

Okay, having stated that – most "expiration dates" on medicine can be greatly extended. The military did a test on this and most medicines don't go bad – they merely lose strength (in many cases, they remain viable long after the date on the package.) Evidently, one exception is aspirin. If the aspirin smells vinegary, toss it out. We save our old medications. You need to do whatever your doctor tells you to do.

Penicillin V Procaine is penicillin – whether it comes with a prescription from your doctor for a human or if it comes from the veterinarian supply house for your goats. Tetracycline is the same whether it is for humans or fish. You just need to learn what dosages and courses of treatment are viable for you. This can usually be calculated by weight but there are other factors that figure in. I am just making you aware of the fact that antibiotics are available. It's up to you to do the proper research to decide if and how you will use them.

Is there a place in your preparations for herbal medicines? I think there could be. This will also require research on your part to identify local plants that can be used. I do *not* recommend buying so called herbal remedies as a way of ensuring you are not "controlled by Big Medicine" in the future. Doing this only trades one supplier for another – not very self-sufficient. I recommend you identify *local* herbs and learn how to prepare them yourself. You will need to research this. I suggest you start at the library and museum. The internet is also a good source. The key here is to get out and do it – don't just read about it.

Supplies
What kind of supplies do you need? Like everything else, this depends on your threat analysis. You will definitely want a comprehensive first aid kid. You will probably want several refills of contents.

You may want to think about long term care. This is where nursing comes in. Patients will need their bed sheets changed and washed. How many sets do you have? Do you have means to wash and dry them in the absence of electricity? What about water? Soap?

Consider obtaining many bandages and dressings – these will have to be changed frequently in a long term crisis situation. Ask a paramedic how much stuff they use on just one car crash – the amounts of bandages, tape, dressings and so on are staggering – and that's just for the initial treatment and packaging. Nursing the injured person back to health will require much more.

Just because you don't know how to use certain materials (i.e. splints) now does not mean you should not purchase them if you find a good deal on them. You may learn how to later. You may find a wandering doctor or nurse who can assist but who has no supplies of their own.

Do not neglect cleaning supplies. You may be cleaning up bodily fluids, having to scrub out buckets people have vomited into and so on. Bleach and ammonia are your friends – just never mix them!

Training

You cannot have too much medical training. Everyone should take a basic first aid course. If you have children, you should know baby and child CPR. Seek out opportunities to learn more. Many communities have volunteer firefighters, community emergency response teams, and so on that would love more volunteers. Not only will you be able to help your community, you will also learn vital new skills.

Join Scouts – yes, you can do it as an adult. Boy Scouts of America has an excellent first aid course in their First Aid merit badge. If you cannot or will not join Scouts, you can at least buy or check out of the library the manual and teach yourself.

Once you receive training you need to continue to practice. Even EMTs, doctors and nurses must earn continuing education credits each year to stay current. You should do likewise. Get out there and practice. Teach others as well.

Hygiene

"The most important aspect of Survival Medicine is proper personal hygiene". We had to memorize that when I attended the SERE (Survival, Evasion, Resistance and Escape) Instructor Qualification Course.

It matters little if you are an evading pilot shot down behind enemy lines, a survival group caught up in some end of the world as we know it situation, or a family living on a self-sufficient homestead – if you fail to maintain basic standards of cleanliness you will make yourself sick.

Your Body

You will need to brush teeth, wash hands frequently and take baths or showers occasionally. I like the idea of alcohol gel hand sanitizer for a quick "wash". Diaper wipes are also a convenient way to take a quick sponge bath.

You can take a sponge bath with just a little bit of water. I used to do it from a canteen cup. Simply heat up a small pot of warm water. Dip a washrag in it and lather it up with some soap – wash your face first then your arm pits and crotch. You could also wash your feet. Just use a little soap and then rinse/wipe off with the washcloth.

Got soap? Know how to make it? Now is as good a time as any to learn. That is beyond the scope of this book but the information is readily available on the Internet. My wife makes lovely lye soap about twice a year – it's just the thing for greasy hands.

Keep your hair covered to prevent crud from getting in it and comb it frequently. Trim and clean under your nails. Always wash your hands before doing three things: cooking, eating, and rendering medical aid. You really don't want to have diarrhea or a flaming infection on top of all the other problems you may be experiencing. Stay clean!

Clothing

You will need to wash your clothes as well. You could use the same water the family took a bath in. I know it sounds gross but our super high personal cleanliness standards will slip a bit in a long term survival situation. When you have to carry buckets of water up from the creek you will learn to take short cuts. And short cuts are okay – just don't forsake bathing completely.

We have scrub boards and an antique clothes washer plunger – it looks like a metal toilet bowl plunger and you use it to agitate the clothes in the soapy water. You can also use a regular toilet bowl plunger to agitate your clothes and wash them in your bath tub, or a five gallon bucket or a wash tub. It helps to have three wash tubs and a big pot. You heat up the water in your pot and pour it into your first wash tub. If the tub is metal you can just heat it up directly. Into this tub you add soap. Then you fill two similar sized tubs with clear water. Scrub and/or agitate clothes in the first tub, then wring them out. Then put them in the second tub for the first rinse. Then wring them out. Then put them in the third tub for final rinse. Then wring them out. That's a lot of water and a lot of wringing.

When I was in South Korea in the 1980s, Korean women would wash on flat rocks in a stream – in the winter as well as summer. Tough women. Solved the wash water problem – but it didn't help the down stream drinking water problem... You will develop a good grip and awesome forearms. Or you could buy a hand cranked wringer. Be advised though, the people who make them are very proud of them (they are expensive). You could also buy a gas powered washing machine. I know they exist but I have no experience with them.

You will need a solar clothes dryer. They are not very expensive. Just buy some clothes line and some clothespins and set it up! If you don't already hang clothes to dry you should start. Believe it or not, there are things to learn here – learn by doing. I love sun dried bath towels. You can hang clothes to dry when it is freezing out. Most of the water will evaporate or freeze as crystals that you knock off by shaking it vigorously. Then you can do the "final dry" inside where it is (hopefully) warmer.

Toilet
Another problem you won't want to deal with but will have to is disposal of human waste. You have several options here. If you are on septic you really don't have to worry about the municipal sewer backing up into your house – like it did a few times while we lived in some third world nation. You could store extra water to put in the toilet tank. You can also use gray water – water you already used to take a bath in, wash clothes in or whatever, to flush your toilet. You can pour it in the tank and use as normal or you can pour it directly into the bowl and it requires a bit less to get the job done. But it can splash...

You could buy a chemical toilet in the camping sections of your local Chinamart – make sure you buy extra chemical and the special toilet paper that requires. You could stock up on plastic bags and have a bucket on hand. I have a friend who has tested a saw dust bucket. You basically do your business I the bucket which contains a layer of saw dust and then cover it with some more saw dust. When it is full, you put in into a pit to decompose. Mind your water source... My friend as tested this device which he built for his fallout shelter and swears it doesn't stink – much.

Another option is to dig an outhouse in the back yard. This last option would probably violate a thousand codes and ordinances where you live – you may wish to check with proper authorities. Or not. Our Y2K plan included digging an outhouse in our suburban back yard inside a storage shed.

Which ever method you use, make sure you wash up afterwards. It may help to suspend an old milk jug near your latrine. Fill it with water and tie an old onion bag containing a bar of soap to the handle with a length of cord. Poke a small hole in the bottom side of the jug and fit it with a carved wooden peg. To use, simply loosen the cap to allow air in and let water dribble out of the bottom hole – lather and rinse.

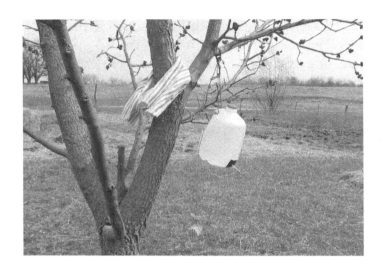

Dishes and Cookware

In a short term emergency it is really nice to have a supply of paper plates, cups and plastic silverware – use and discard. You may use it for fuel for your next cooking fire. When I lived in a tropical country, the natives, instead of dishes, would eat off of banana leaves – in restaurants! It sure made the dishwasher's job easier.

Eventually though you will have pots and plates to deal with. One way to clean them is the "three pot method". As you are sitting down to eat, place a pot of water on the fire/stove/grill to heat up. When ready to wash up, pour about a third of the water into another basin or pot and then add cold water to the second container to fill it up. Fill a third container with cold water. Pour some soap into the hot water pot. Wash your dish in this hot soapy water. Rinse it in the warm clear water and give it a final rinse the cold clear water. Some folks add a bit of bleach to the final rinse.

It helps if you wash the cleanest plates first and work your way down to the dirty stuff. It helps if people "lick their plates clean" – they can do it with a piece of bread. When done washing, empty the basins in the following manner: 1) Pour out the hot soapy water; 2) pour the warm clear water into the now empty pot and then pour the cold clear water into the formerly warm container. Put the cold clear water container away. Swish the warm water around the original pot and pour it out. Swish the cold water around the "warm" container and then pour it into the hot pot. Swish and pour out. Now all three have been rinsed with clean water.

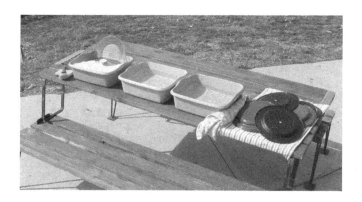

Camping

Your family should be comfortable camping. Being able to do this without a lot of added drama could help immeasurably if you were forced to flee your home during times of crisis. Basic outdoor skills and woodsmanship should form the core of your survival skills. If you have not yet camped as a family, I highly recommend it. The first few times will feel strange -

you won't know what to bring and so you will bring too much. Great! Just as long as you get out and enjoy yourself.

Start easy - go to the nearest state park and camp there. Bring along charcoal to cook on, some chairs, a cooler of drinks. Go and spend a Saturday and then sleep out. You'll thank me when you get home.

Camping as a family enables you all to learn so much: delegation of responsibility and chores, organization, planning, packing and unpacking, communication and so on. You also learn how to make yourself comfortable without "all the comforts of home". You will learn how to cook without a stove, how to clean up, how make yourself comfortable on the ground. You will learn that you do not *need* a climate controlled environment.

You will learn what gear works and what gear does not. You will find things you like, things that suit you – not just something you read about. After you have camped several times and acquired the basic equipment you will discover that your family can handle a three-day power outage without missing a beat.

What will you need? Well, again, it will depend on you and your family but my family finds the following items useful:

Tents
We like tents you can stand up in. It makes it easy to get dressed and does not feel claustrophobic. Sometimes we even bring a low folding chair in there.

My wife and I sleep in an 8x8x six feet high tent. When they were very young, our children slept with us. As they got older we moved them into a similarly sized tent. Then our youngest grew up and she and her sister would sleep in the "kids' tent" and our son would pitch his own backpacker tent.

No one likes a leaky tent. Make sure you seam seal your tent. Wherever the stitches are on your tent there are holes that go all the way through. Holes that will allow water to get in. Seam seal is this liquid glue stuff you can buy at any camping store and you simply apply it to all of your seams prior to going camping. You will have to set your tent up in the back yard to do this correctly. You should set it up beforehand anyway so you know how to do it.

After you seam seal it, you will want to add additional waterproofing. Yes, your rain fly is supposedly waterproof. Uh-huh... I used to spray a silicon waterproofing compound on my tent but it would wear off rather quickly. Then a buddy of mine, Mike Hawk, showed me a cool trick: use deck seal. Yep, the stuff you put on your wood deck. Just paint it on your fly and the parts of your tent that extend below your fly. Man, this works well. If you use deck stain as opposed to just clear sealant you will even subdue the colors a bit.

Ground Cloths
We just use poly tarps. They protect the floor of your tent from any sharp things you missed when setting the tent up. Make sure you tuck your tarps all the way under your tent so water flowing off the tent hits the ground and not your tarp. If it hits your tarp, it

will flow under the tent and find a way up through
your floor.

Folding Chairs
The normal sized ones really work well when you
want to take a load off your feet. Everyone should
have their own chair. If you camp with other families
(which is fun), you should paint a certain colored
stripe or something on all your gear so it's easy to see
what is yours and what is not.

Lanterns
We hang a kerosene lantern up at night before
everyone goes to bed. This way, family members can
become oriented as soon as they pop their head out
of the tent and if they walk away from the tent site to
"use a tree" they can easily find their way back.

We also give the kids a battery powered lantern to use
in their tent – it makes them a lot more comfortable
getting dressed and undressed and allows them to play
inside if the weather is bad.

Cooking Utensils
We typically make simple meals when we camp. Fry
burgers, bacon, and eggs in a frying pan. You may
want a big pot for boiling water, cooking hotdogs,
making pasta, soup, etc. Another pot can be handy
so you can have two going at once. Hot pads, grills
(we found ours in an abandoned stove), gloves, long
handled spatulas – all work in the utensil category.
You will not want any plastic if you are cooking over
fire (and I encourage you to do so) as plastic will melt.

You already read about Dutch ovens and all the tools
that go along with them but for a quick review: you

will want a lid lifter, leather gloves, and a shovel at a minimum.

Coolers
At least one for drinks at least and as many as you need for the food you bring. Sometimes on long term campouts we have to run to town for more ice. My girls never seem to mind the trip.

Water Cans
Some campsites have water and others do not. Those with water do not typically have a spigot at every campsite. So you will need something to haul water in. It's nice to have a couple 5 gallon cans of water in your kitchen area while camping.

Bins and Bags
We carry stuff in Rubbermaid Tote bins. We have one marked "Kitchen" which contains the tools, pots, pans, clean up stuff, tablecloth and so on. We have others that hold miscellaneous tools like a hammer and some nails, wire, cordage, tape, or Lanterns and fuel, or radio gear and batteries, and so on.

We limit every person to one large and one small bag when we are car camping. For large bags kit bags or duffels work well and this is where we store the bulk of our clothing. Each person uses the small bag (typically a day pack) to hold toiletries, personal items, and things they want to be able to access quickly.

If you keep your gear organized and in one place it makes it fairly simple to go camping on a whim – or bug out. Just grab the "camp bins", coolers, tentage, sleeping bags and personal bags and you can go. Get your food at home or on the way.

Firearms

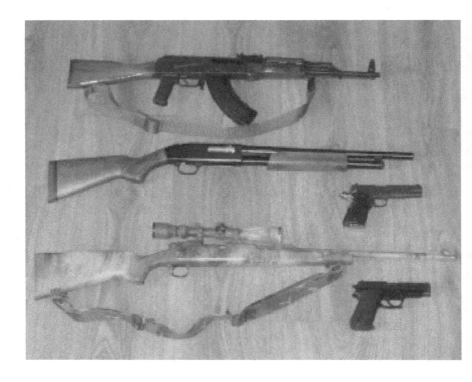

You are ultimately responsible for the security of your family. Providing this may entail the use of firearms. Children can be taught proper use and safety in this area - it is up to you to make the final decision. For those with children, I highly recommend Massad Ayoob's book <u>Gunproof your Children!</u> I'll tell you right up front though – if you are going to have accessible firearms in your home, you need disciplined children. Your kids – your call.

We really need firearms for two purposes: hunting and defense. Guns are cool, guns can be shiny, and guns impart some weird sense of power to many people.

Whatever. They are tools. Just that.
We determined what firearms we wanted and
purchased them a long time ago. You don't need
many. You should have the basics though.

Pump Shotgun

This is the basic firearm that should be required by
law to be maintained in every home. I recommend a
pump because they are simple to learn to operate,
they are less complex in operation, and they are less
expensive than semi-autos. Single and double barrels
may suffice for hunting but they are not ideal for
defensive purposes due to the lack of ammunition
capacity.

Normally for those on a budget (and who isn't?)
and with smaller wives I recommend a 20 gauge. At
household distances a 20 gauge is just as effective
as a 12 gauge but with significantly reduced recoil. I
also recommend a youth model. Youth models have
shorter buttstocks and longer fore ends which make
them easier to handle by those with short arms.
Those with big arms have very little problems shooting
them. Conversely, smaller people have a difficult time
shooting shotguns that are too big for them.

I really like Mossberg 500 "combo models". I
recommend this shotgun for a few reasons. First,
Mossberg makes the least expensive decent pump
shotgun. No, it's not as famous as some others will
cool logos. That logo on the side will cost you at least
an additional $100 and you won't get the spare barrel
and chokes you get with a Mossy. That's right – the
combo package comes with an 18.25 inch barrel ideal
for defensive purposes and a longer, vent-ribbed barrel

complete with three screw-in choke tubes so you can use it to hunt just about whatever you want. It also comes with a really sexy pistol grip. I tell everyone to sell the pistol grip at the next gun show and use the money to buy more ammo.

Now, I could write a book just on shotguns and some day I may, but to keep this manageable let me conclude by saying a pump shotgun as described is an extremely versatile weapon: you can defend the homestead and hunt everything from squirrels to turkey to geese to bears with them. If you don't own one you should really just stop reading and go buy one. Now.

Deer Rifle
We are describing a bolt action rifle of approximately .30 caliber with a scope. Now I am not big on goo-gaws and gadgets and the latest trend in gear. That is my deer rifle up there and to the uninitiated it looks "high speed". I assure you it is not. It is just a base-model Remington 700 in .308 with a Bushnell scope and about $3 worth of Krylon spray paint. You can pick something like this up (minus the paint job) at most Chinamarts for less than $600 as of this printing.

Now entire Internet forums are dedicated to firearms. There you will find folks who argue incessantly about this detail or that. I'm a basic guy. I use basic gear. If that gear works, I'm not usually in a hurry to replace it. Take my deer rifle. It is not special. It doesn't have a synthetic stock or pillar bedding, an adjustable trigger, or any other gadgets. My scope is a basic off the shelf model that I paid $32 for. You can spend four times as much on a deer rifle set up. But you know what? I have killed about 30 deer with that rifle. I never miss. And that basic, low budget rifle is capable of shooting better than most people who pick it up. It does no good to buy a rifle that will shoot sub-minute of angle groups if you are not a sub-minute of angle shooter. And the vast majority is not. Also, to hunt deer, one does not need that kind of accuracy – you need to hit a fairly large target area to put a deer down. Buy a basic rifle, learn to shoot it well. Spend you money on ammo and training and only then consider upgrading to a better rifle.

Why buy a deer rifle? Because you can shoot big things far away with it. That could be a deer, or a cow, or a crazed zombie mutant. Much better to shoot them way over there than in the living room. 'Nuff said.

Pistol
Every adult should have a handgun. Every adult should be armed all the time – you don't get to pick when Trouble is coming to visit. You will not be carrying a shotgun or rifle around with you 24/7. There is a cutesy phrase that circulates amongst the gun culture that says, "A pistol is to fight your way back to the rifle you should not have set down in the first place." Yeah...

Get a handgun. Here I will once again enter into the fray: As long as it is .38 Special or better, it really doesn't matter what caliber you get. I have a friend that shoots 9mm. I used to tease him unmercifully. I'd say things like, "9mm is a fine caliber – my daughters shoot it. My wife even used to shoot it until she moved up to .45". I don't want to enter the caliber wars so I'll just stick with what I said - .38 Special or better. I will also say that it really doesn't matter if it's a wheel gun (revolver) or a semi-automatic. Just get one you will feel comfortable toting around all day, every day. And once you get your handgun – go get trained in its use. First learn how to shoot safely and accurately. This is basic handgun instruction. Then go learn how to fight with it – you will pay good money for this instruction and if you ever need to use your handgun for real it will have been worth every penny.

Battle Rifle

You may never need it. But if you do – you will be so glad you have had one, trained with it, and gotten very familiar with its use. I don't think you should waste anytime in obtaining one either. It's just a matter of time before someone tries to infringe your right to keep and bear...

Again, I will not enter the fray on which type to buy. I will just say this – get a platform that closely mimics a proven military arm. AR15, AK47, M1A, FAL, etc, etc. Basically you want a weapon that is robust, that fires a proven cartridge, and that takes magazines so that it can be reloaded quickly.

I chose the Mossberg 500 because it is the least expensive decent pump gun. For the same reasons, I recommended that budget minded folks buy an AK47 clone. Of all the decent "assault rifles" it is the cheapest. And for the record, I am not a huge AK fan personally. But I am also not trying to build an armory over night with limited funds. When you get your rifle, get a bunch of magazines for it. Get real magazines – not some cheap knock off. Having twelve would not be too many. Not by a long shot.

Closing Thoughts

Some survivalist writers are very enamored with the .22. They say .22 ammunition will be the new currency after the collapse. I don't think so. I just don't think there will be that much left to shoot at after most folks use up the .22 ammo they already have. Yes, a lot of people use .22s. It's just that I do not. I have shot squirrels with them but I much prefer shotguns. If you want this or any other firearm though- please don't let me stand in your way – by all means obtain one!

So those are the basics according to Joe. For those with no guns at all, I recommend you go out and get this battery as quickly as possible. We are potentially just two days (at any given time) away from total chaos. Gabe Suarez said something that keeps resonating through my mind – "The only thing harder than preparing is having to explain why you didn't".

Is this an ideal battery? Of course not. It is a working one though. It would be better if one would standardize weapons and calibers. For example, one could get a deer rifle in .308 and then choose a .308 battle rifle such as an FAL, or MIA. Ideally, a family would purchase identical pistols or at least caliber, for the adults to use as well. It would be great if every member of the family had a complete set of the above weapons – all identical.

But in the end, your family is not a military unit – you don't *need* to be standardized. You won't be shooting a million rounds at mutant zombies over the course of your lifetime – but you could very conceivably have to go through several magazines at some point in your life.

Time is getting short. I hope that you never have to sit down and cry because you spent your money on big screen televisions and electronics instead of basic gear – basic gear like a basic battery.

Ammunition

You will obviously need ammunition for your firearms. I think you should go ahead and get a life time supply just as soon as you can afford to. What is a lifetime supply though?

I came up with a "comfort level" for ammo based on my yearly hunting usage. For example last year I fired 6 rounds out of my deer rifle - 3 to confirm zero and one for each deer I killed. I fired a lot more shotgun ammo. I occasionally shoot recreationally (IDPA, plinking) and so I keep some ammo on hand for that. When I use a box I buy a box. If I see a great deal on bulk ammo for one of my firearms I may buy some. One thing I've started doing is buying cleaning supplies every time I buy ammo.

A number you will hear bandied about when survivalist ammunition is discussed is 10,000 rounds.

10,000 Rounds

Long, long ago, in a land far away I was preparing to brief some big shots a plan that entailed me and some scary friends of mine going to a scary place to do scary things. The problem was, we had no podium. Priorities, ya know? So we made a podium out of AK47 ammo crates. The only comment one of the VIPs had after the brief was, "nice podium". *Suits...*

Since that time I have sometimes fantasized about buying enough AK ammo to build my own podium – that would be about 6 or 7 cases I reckon. Why? Nostalgia I guess. But I never did buy that much ammo.

The Experts Say...

Spend enough time on the Internet surfing survivalist forums or read enough survivalist literature and you will eventually get to the part where folks talk about how much ammo one will need in an end of the world scenario. One number frequently tossed out there is 10,000 rounds.

"You will need 10,000 rounds per main battle rifle." Why 10,000? Why not 7,000? Why not 14,000? I suspect that, like my whimsical podium, it's just a nice round number. I doubt anyone ever sat down and said, "Let's see here, I will expend 300 rounds per fire fight and I will get into this many firefights over the next 5 years..." C'mon!

It's shiny

People fear or fantasize (take your pick) about not being able to get the ammo they need "when the time comes". Operative word – "they". See, they are not stockpiling ammo for some resistance cell. They view this as personal ammo for them and their immediate family – most of who are typically not on board.

Ammo is one of those things that is easy to purchase, it stacks nicely and it's shiny. It does not require a lot of work or sweat or thought to amass a big ol' pile of it. It makes people feel good like a bowl of chocolate ice cream makes me feel good. But if I thought about it before I dug into that bowl, I'd realize that the several hundred useless calories I was about to consume would have to be burned off by endless burpees or miles of forest trail – or it will turn to fat. But I don't think about that when I'm chowing down.

I don't think folks who toss around big numbers for *required* amounts of ammo are thinking too deeply either.

The Other Stuff

If one assumes that one is going to expend 10,000 rounds of ammo (because why buy it if one isn't going to use it?) then one must assume he is going to break some parts. Extractors, pins, handguards. Less common is the call for stockpiling spare parts – it's not as sexy. But we do see some talk of that. Something we never see is cleaning supplies. If you can't get ammo at the store – where will you get cleaning supplies? Most guns get pretty dirty after 1,000 rounds. If you are fighting like your life depends on it, you will want a clean weapon right? *"We'll use rags and motor oil."* Uh-huh. Cleaning supplies are REALLY not sexy. So no one wants enough patches and CLP and spare rods and so on.

But the thing that really gets me going is the lack of medical preparations. You see, any scenario that one could envision that would require expending 10,000 rounds of "main battle rifle ammo" would necessarily entail bad guys who shoot back. We ain't shooting cardboard here. This is where brows start to furrow. This is where the fantasy starts to unravel. That same scenario probably has you with people you love and care about – buddies, family members and so on. If you shoot 10,000 rounds at bad guys - they are gonna shoot at least that many back at you. Someone you care about is going to get hit. And live. At least initially.

It's all fun and games 'til someone gets an eye poked out
Have you ever seen a gunshot wound? Have you ever seen someone shot through the belly? They live. They hurt. They are very unhappy – big sad face. So, after we win the fire fight with our superior fighting skills... we have to deal with Bob, or Sally, or little Ashley.

We are talking skills and supplies. First aid, Advanced Trauma Life Support, blow out kits, IVs and so on. That's to get them through the initial stage. Then there is the long term care and nursing required to fight infection, repair torn up bodies and so on. It takes an enormous amount of gauze and tape and tubing and wrapping to deal with one gunshot wound. It takes a whole lot more to nurse them back to health.

So, for those recommending buying 10,000 rounds of ammo for each MBR, why do we not hear about or see similar recommendations for medical gear? Where is their field hospital complete with cots, and sheets, and pans and instruments and more bandages than you can shake a stick at? Where is the staff or the personal training undertaken to handle such situations? It's not there.

Because it's not easy and it's not sexy. It's not easy to think about a loved one dying over the course of a week from a gut shot. It's not easy to acquire the skills for dealing with these things – or recruiting those who can. Bandages don't come in flat black with

Velcro or in the latest digi-cam pattern.

Guys and Gals – please think this through.

Should you store up some ammunition? Absolutely.
Do you need 10,000 rounds?
You tell me – are you well rounded? Have you taken
care of everything else?

Storage

I store my ammo in military surplus ammo cans. They
are inexpensive and easily obtained at gun shows. If
you do purchase a lot of ammo, give some thought
to where you are going to store it. When fire hits
ammunition it starts "popping" as the powder gets hot
and burns/explodes. The bullets do not go whizzing
all over the place contrary to what you see in the
movies. Because the round is not contained in firearm
chamber when it pops there is not enough pressure
to send the bullet anywhere. But it does make noise.
And not all firefighters know about it being relatively
harmless so they may back off and let your house
burn until the ammo stops "cooking off".

Keep your ammo dry and not too hot and it will last
for decades if not longer. Don't keep it in your attic
and if you do keep it in your basement, make sure it
is in waterproof containers (like ammo cans) and has
desiccant in there with it.

Tools

Survivalists are self-sufficient. We do things for
ourselves. To do many things we will need the proper
tools. The best advice I ever got on tools was – "When

you need a tool – buy one, don't borrow it." That is sound advice if you think you will ever use that tool again. I got this advice when I was trying to build a set of book shelves for my ever-expanding library. The first set of shelves I built was just terrible – they wobbled badly from side to side. The friend who gave me that advice showed up to help me and the first thing he said was – "you have no back on those shelves – let's build one." He proceeded to measure my sad shelves, lay a piece of plywood on his sawhorses, pulled a chalk line out of his carpenter's belt, snapped a line and then cut that board with a circular saw. It took him about 5 minutes. The only tool I had like all the ones he had just used was a tape measure and mine was only 10' long whereas his was 25' long.

My buddy then told me to screw the back on while he set about working on the new shelves. *"Ah ha"*, I thought, *"THIS is something I can do – I have a screw driver."*

I had done many projects where I screwed in several wood screws in a row. I had a Phillips head screwdriver and I really appreciated the rounded handle because it didn't blister my palm quite as fast as the more square shaped ones would when I had to drive more than about ten screws at a time. My buddy wasn't paying attention at first and as I was setting the third of what would end up being about 20 screws he shook his head and went back out to his truck.

He returned with a cordless drill that had a cross slot bit and a box of deck screws. "Here, use this", he said. After he showed me how to use it I got to work and oh, did a BIG light bulb switch on in my head! "I have *got* to get me one of these!" And that is when I discovered the need for tools – proper tools.

The survivalist living in suburbia will require different tools than one living on a farm. But even our suburban brethren should have enough to build a bookcase, repair a toilet, and construct a closet or small shed. The following tools should get you started. I like giving tools for wedding presents. I mean, what is really more practical – a wok or a cordless drill? When you buy tools you really don't have to buy top of the line – but you shouldn't buy the cheapest Chinese junk either. Look around, talk to people who use tools – they'll give you decent advice.

The Basic Tool Box
These initial tools should be kept in a plastic tool box and stored inside the home. Always put your tools back when you are done using them and you will have them when you need them. This kit makes a great present for a young adult setting up house for the first time.
Plastic tool box – Get one bigger than you think you'll need – you will add stuff to it.

Sharpie – Start right from the get-go labeling every tool you own with your name. You will find yourself at a your buddy's house having a "bookshelf building party" and when it's time to go you will quickly discover that your friends bought their tools the same place you bought yours – they will all look the same but some will be in better condition than others. Some people will paint all of their tools with some obnoxious color like orange. My son bought a whole set of tools and the previous owner had hit every tool with a splash of orange spray paint. Others get fancy and devise a color scheme of stripes – for example: White, Orange, White – with which they label all their tools. This makes it easy to identify at a distance. Someday I will do this with Black, Yellow, Black but I have a lot of more pressing chores to do now so a Sharpie just has to suffice.

Pencils – You will be making notes, marking measures, drawing lines and other innumerable tasks. Pens run out of ink at the worst time. Pencils can be easily re-sharpened. You will need more than one because you will always set it down and forget it.

Ruler – You will need a ruler to draw straight lines, make simple measurements and so on. One of those kid's plastic rulers with the three holes to fit in a notebook will be fine.

Small notebook – When you build things you make notes. You may be measuring the shelf you want in the dining room and go out to the garage to cut it. If you don't write it down you will forget your data. You will also make lists. It is very annoying to drive 20 miles to the nearest hardware or home improvement store, buy your needed items and return another 20 miles only to remember that you forgot the one really important item which is required to complete the project.

Knives – Some folks get by with just a utility knife but I like a regular pocket knife also. You will sharpen your pencils, cut cord, carve a smidge off the end of that board, cut tile, scribe a line, and so on. Definitely get the utility knife and an extra pack of blades.

167

Screwdrivers – To change the blade on your utility knife you will need a flat tip screw driver. You will need screwdrivers for lots of things. Get about three or four sizes of both flat tip and cross tip (Phillips) screwdrivers. Spend some money here - the handles will break on the cheap ones. I like Craftsman for most of my basic tools. Use your screwdrivers for screws – not to stir paint, chisel wood, or as pry bars.

Pliers – These are a valuable tool and you will use them frequently. You need at least one slip-joint pliers but two sizes is handier. You use them to hold nuts while screwing in a bolt, grabbing hard to grab things (like the head of a finishing nail in the wall) and so on. You will also want a pair of needle nosed pliers to grab those small things. Needle nose pliers also have a wire cutter built in.

Claw Hammer – You need a hammer to pound nails for hanging pictures, pull nails out of the wall and so on. Get one the smallest adult in your household is comfortable using – they come in a variety of sizes. It is truly amazing how many different types of hammers there are.

Tape Measure – Get a 10 to 15 foot long tape measure for your tool box. It will handle most chores in the house.

Socket Wrench – These are amazing tools for loosening and tightening nut and bolts. They ratchet so you do not have to continuously reposition it as you are spinning the nut around and around. These are great for putting bunk beds together! Do yourself a favor and spend some money here. Cheap socket sets don't

last long. You want one where the "switch" is metal –
the plastic ones wear out quickly. You will want both
metric and inch pattern sockets.

Tape – Get a roll each of duct tape (it rules the world!),
masking tape, and black electric tape. Don't buy
cheap electric tape – it won't stick long. You will find
yourself using lots of masking tape for marking things.
You can make notes on it and when you remove the
tape it doesn't leave a residue like duct tape will.

Nails – Get a small box of finishing nails and another
of 3" common nails. You will use these primarily to
hang pictures and what not in the house and it's just
easier to have them in the tool box when you need
them.

That is the basic kit. Everyone should have this in
their home. When you are first starting out, you
will not have duplicates of tools so when you need
a hammer in the garage, you will have to go and get
your basic tool box. Eventually though, you will start
acquiring spares and you will keep tools where you
primarily use them.

Light Construction Tools
Your basic tool box will see you through most in house
repairs and duties. But you are not done yet, you still
need more tools to take care of light construction –
things like building shelves, making a bench, a planter
and so on. These tools are typically larger and don't fit
in a kitchen drawer very well so most folks keep them
in the garage or workshop.
Hammer – If you don't already own a framing hammer
– buy one. Due to the length, leverage and weight,
they are awesome when you have to drive a six penny

nail into a 2x4. You can even do rough measuring for 16" on center studs with this tool.

25' Tape Measure – You will need this when you are doing serious work. It's a bit large for normal day to day stuff around the house and that's why we don't keep one in the tool box.

Circular Saw – These are electric and are awesome when it's time to cut several 2x4s or a piece of plywood. I have had a Black and Decker for over 20 years and it's still going strong.

Electric Drill – These are great for doing medium duty work around the workshop. Buy a couple sets of bits – some for wood, some for metal and keep them all together in their own tool box.

Cordless Drill – How I ever lived without one, I'll never know. I use mine primarily for driving screws. They typically come with two batteries and a charger. Go ahead and buy an extra battery now. I went for years with a 12 volt drill and finally made the switch to an 18 volt drill. The 18 volt is larger, heavier and has a lot more torque. My wife thinks it's too heavy. If you can wield it, go big early. If money is not a problem, buy a 12 volt for the basic tool box and the larger one for the shop. Buy several screw bits to go with it. You'll save battery power if you pre-drill your screw holes with an electric drill and drive them with the cordless drill.

50' Extension Cord – Get a heavy duty one designed for outdoor use. You may want two of them.
Cross Cut saw – Get one of those shorter ones about two feet long for when you just have a quick saw job and don't feel like hooking up the circular saw.

Hack Saw – This is for cutting metal but will also work on plastic. Get a couple packs of blades when you pick one up. You can mount the blade teeth facing in if you need to in order to reach a tight spot.

Carpenter's Square – This looks like a big metal L-shaped ruler. You will use it more than you think. Almost anything you build will need to be "square" and this is the tool for that.

Speed Square – This looks like a triangle and the more I use mine, the more I like it. Get a light weight one – plastic is fine.

Saw Horses – You can make a set, buy components to make a set or buy some light weight folding plastic ones – that's what I did and they work okay. For heavy work you really want more substantial saw horses. I went for years without these, balancing my work on trash cans, tables, the pickup tail gate – you name it. Saw horses make a big difference.

Levels – Get a 3 foot long one and the folding "speed level" which measures for level in several directions simultaneously. The latter is great for setting poles in the ground.

Pry Bars – Get a long crow bar which is basically round in cross section and a short little handy one typically formed from flat stock. You may end up keeping the little one in your tool box – it's great for pulling nails, removing molding and trim and so on. *Bolt Cutters* – When you need to cut that pesky lock, chain, or even – bolt! Get a pair about 3 feet long and spend some money here – the cheap ones break quickly.

171

Tool Belt – These are so important when you are working on a project. They save you an incredible amount of time looking for stuff, climbing up and down the ladder and so on. You have to train yourself to use it correctly – always put your tool back in its proper place on the belt or you will end up looking for it. My wife and I each have our own set up how we like it. There are pockets for nails, screws, and what not; a place to hold your pencil, clip on your tape measure, sling your hammer and just about anything else you want.

Step ladder – You will use this a lot. Be careful when setting it up and don't teeter-totter on the top "step". *Protective Gear* – Get some clear protective glasses, leather gloves, and hearing protectors. Use them! The gloves and ear muffs will hang nicely from your belt on snap links. You will have to cut a hole in the gauntlet portion of your gloves.

Outdoor Tools
You will need tools to work outside, build gardens, level ground for your dog house –whatever.

Shovels – A long handled shovel will save your back from a lot of bending over. I don't like the fancy ones with neoprene sleeves on the handle. Just get a plain old shovel. D-handled shovels are shorter but sometimes you need a short handle so go ahead and get one now. We keep one in each vehicle. *Wheelbarrow* – Haul dirt, rocks, mulch, groceries, the kids... It's worthwhile to investigate no-flat tires.

Dirt Rake – You'll want one for your garden. It works for spreading gravel also.

Hoe – If you garden in the traditional way you will need one for weed control. Get a long handled one to save your back. Keep it sharp! Works on snakes, too.

Axe – Whether you have a fireplace or wood stove or not – you will eventually need an axe. You don't need a $100 Swedish axe but you don't want some cheap Chinese junk one either. I have grown fond of fiberglass handles because they don't break as easy when you miss...

Mill Bastard File and Carborundum Stone – For keeping your axe and hoe sharp. I use them on my shovels too.
100' of Stout Rope – Get manila or good nylon rope – not the cheap poly stuff. You will use rope a lot –especially if you have it. The easiest way to keep the ends from fraying is to tape it off with duct tape. If you are going to cut it, tape it first and then cut through the tape. If it's nylon, you can melt the ends after cutting.

Pulleys – To fit your rope. It is amazing what you can lift with mechanical advantage.

Sledge Hammers – Sometimes you need a bigger hammer. Get a short handled one around 2 pounds and a full sized one. My wife has a 6-pound sledge and I have an 8-pound one.

Splitting Maul and Wedges – If you heat with wood you will want these tools. Get at least three wedges. I like fiberglass handles on my mauls.

Communications

Having the ability to communicate with your family and friends in dangerous times could make the difference between surviving and perishing. The options for communication are many and we will explore a few of them now.

Cell Phones

Every member of your family who travels away from the house by themselves should have a cell phone. In fact anytime a group leaves the home at least one member of that group should have a functioning cell phone. If you live out away from the bright city lights (and you should) you may occasionally experience spotty service. Sometimes when a voice message will not get through a text message will. Also, texting uses up less battery power than talking. I learned this from my children. Cell phones cannot be your only means of communication though because during times of crisis the cells get overloaded with everyone trying to communicate and so they no longer work.

FRS

Family Radio Service radios are very good over short distances (about a mile or so) and straight line with no large intervening mountains or cityscape. They are basically small walkie-talkies. My wife got our first set when Motorola put them out and I think they were $98 then. You can at times find a set now for less than $10. These work very well when convoying, hunting (although you need to check your game regulations as to whether or not they are legal for this in your area), and all manner of outdoor activities. Problems arise when you get into a very crowded place like an

amusement park and all the channels get clogged up.
They go through batteries fairly quickly so you will
need a good supply or a few sets of rechargeable ones
and a means to do so. Solar can be a good deal in the
right environment.

GMRS

Ground Mobile Radio Service radios look like FRS
radios but they have more power and transmit
further. On a good day, if the stars align and
everything is perfect you can squeeze up to five miles
out of these little transceivers. But under normal
conditions if you get 2 miles out of it you are doing
well. You are supposed to apply for an inexpensive
license before you use (but not before you purchase)
these radios but I really don't think most people
bother. You should probably consult your lawyer for
advice in this area.

CBs

Citizen Band radios used to be in every 18-wheeler
in the land. Most still have one, but anymore people
communicate with cell phones and laptops. We have
hand held and vehicle mounted CBs that we use
whenever we travel any kind of distance by car. The
range on these depends on antennas, power, and line
of sight but a couple of miles is usually not much of
a problem. Because they are falling out of favor – it is
now easier to find clear channels on which to operate.
A couple hand held CBs would make a good addition
to a group's supplies.

Ham

Much to the dismay of several of my ham friends, I
am not a ham radio operator. To operate a ham radio
you need to pass a written test and pay a fee. The test

is not too hard. If you operate a ham radio without a license you are breaking the law and hams in general take a pretty dim view of those who do. They actually try to direction find and catch scofflaws at which point I think the offender can receive a hefty fine.

 Anyway there are 2-meter ham radios that look like walkie-talkies and are good for tens of miles and even further if you can tap into a repeater tower (these towers are known to hams). And there are larger HF (high frequency) sets that can conceivably reach around the world. You learn how to do these things when you study for your test and work with other hams. A lot of your performance depends on what type of antennas you use.

Scanners
You can buy tabletop, vehicle mounted and hand held scanners to continuously search a broad array of frequencies. You can program them to scan your local fire, EMS and police (where it's not scrambled) and you can program them to scan the other popular frequencies in your area. Be aware that others can do this as well and could very well be picking up on your transmissions. Scanners are one good way to maintain situational awareness in your area of operations. You should have a couple.

Internet
Let's face it – the Internet is an awesome way to communicate with others. You can do so in many ways from instant messaging to e-mail, to forums. There is even a way to work a ham radio over the internet although I am not qualified to discuss "packet radio".

Key Points

The key points to remember about communication are these:

Most electronic means are not secure – If you transmit, someone is obviously picking it up. That someone may be someone you don't know about or don't want to be listening in. Please keep this in mind before you *push to talk*.

Effective communication requires training – If you plan on using radios during a crisis it would be a good idea for everyone to practice and be very familiar with they chosen systems before the crisis occurs.

Have multiple redundant systems – If you are going to depend on an FRS for each member of your family you may want to purchase spares now. Things break. Often when you need them the most. It's a good idea with communications just like in other areas not to put all your eggs in one basket or all your trust in one system. Be familiar with and capable of using alternate means of communication.

Be discrete – Use the least power and broadcast over the narrowest range needed to accomplish the communication. You don't want the world listening in. This could be as simple as using low power settings when they will work, to posting messages on restricted internet forums.

Antennas are important – They are important to getting the most range out of any given system and can also be set up and used to somewhat mask your transmissions to keep others from listening in.

Have a "No Commo" plan – Have a plan for what everyone is to do in the event communication stops or fails altogether. It could be as simple as a physical link up point or as complicated as continuing on with certain pre-planned actions.

References

My family has an extensive library and most of the books are "how to" or instructional texts. Periodically local libraries will have sales at which you can sometimes obtain very good books at ridiculous prices. I went to one one time where you could fill a grocery bag with books for a dollar. I have a lot of information saved on my computer but I never trust that medium of storage – too much can go wrong for a technology dinosaur like me. I like instead to have printed pages.

You should read your reference material. Most of you are probably wondering what I'm talking about but I have met more than one person with extensive "survivalist libraries" who had not read most of the books. As if simply having the books imparted knowledge by osmosis or something. The usual excuse is, "I'll have it later if I need it." Better to read it now so at least you are familiar with the subject. Now I will admit, I do have some books I have not (yet) read. Books on subjects like ham radios. Subjects I fully expect to delve into later. Just make sure your read books outnumber your unread ones.

Your library should have some kind of order to it. I do not have a numbering system but I do have my own system and I know where every book goes. My library begins with medical books, flows through to veterinary titles, then animals in general to trees and plants and gardening, to outdoor activities books to wilderness survival and on and on through subjects like lock picking, Native Americans, religious studies and so on. The point being this – when you need a particular reference, you should be able to locate it quickly and efficiently.

As your library grows, people will want to borrow your books. You should establish some kind of system to keep track of who has what - even if it is nothing more than a piece of paper on the last shelf. If you don't, you will forget who you lent a particularly good book to, and they will forget that it is yours.

A list of some of what I consider my better titles is located at Appendix H.

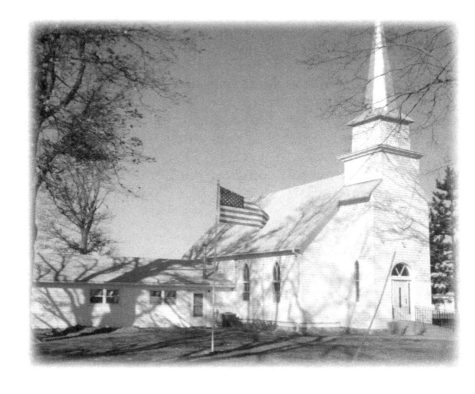

Conclusion

The motto of my company, Viking Services LLC is *Prepared Americans for a Strong America.*

Every American (and indeed, every person - regardless of nationality) who prepares to meet potential problems, difficulties, disasters, and catastrophes is one less person government officials need to be concerned about during a time when they will have more needing help than resources available to meet those needs. If every person and family took the basic steps outlined in this book we would be a stronger nation.

Now that you have finished it, I pray that, if you have not already done so – you go back through this book again and dog ear pages, scrawl in the margins, make lists and then resolve to put this information to use.

Now.

Time is short. Time is our most precious resource – once we use it, we can never get it back.

I would like to invite you to our website hub: <u>www. VikingPreparedness.com</u> . There you will find forums in which you may ask questions and discuss preparedness issues as well as my blog on preparedness and security matters and our ever changing school website.

You are obviously interested in preparedness and have at least some concern for your future – why else would you have waded through this book? Survival preparedness - It's important. But it is not the most important thing. See, this book has been about your and your loved ones' physical survival. What I'd like to leave you with concerns something much more important.

We all want to live long and prosperous lives. But despite our efforts, we are all very likely going to die. What comes next is more important. I am talking about eternal life. This life is so very, very short compared with eternity.

If you don't already know Him, I would like to invite you to meet Jesus Christ. He was and is the Son of God. He was born of a virgin, lived a perfect and sinless life and then was killed for all of our sins. He died and then rose again and now sits at the right hand of the Father and is coming again someday to judge those who are alive and those who are dead.

We are all sinners. Any bit of past sin will keep us from the presence of God. But the cool thing is, Jesus took all those sins upon Himself – our sins are paid for! All we must do is accept this free gift and it's as if we never sinned at all. Accept Jesus. Just pray for Him to come into your life and be your Lord and He'll take it from there!

Jesus said, *"Behold, I stand at the door, and knock: if any man hear my voice, and open the door, I will come in to him, and will sup with him, and he with me."*

My prayer is that you do hear His voice and open that door.

I want you and your family to live. I want you to live in the here and now and I want to see you in the great beyond.

I'll see ya out there!

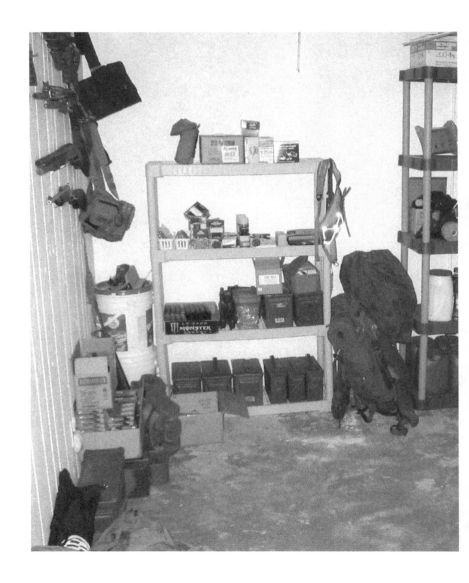

APPENDICES

A. The Basics

Keep these items in one general location of your home so that you can access them all easily. Rubbermaid Tote bins, 5 gallon buckets and duffel bags make good containers for the various items.

Water and Food

Water – 14 gallons per person
Food – two weeks worth of food requiring minimum preparation
Can opener if needed
Paper plates,
Plastic utensils

Hygiene

Paper towels
Garbage bags
Wet wipes
Soap
Chlorine bleach
Hand sanitizer
Feminine hygiene needs
Diapers and wipes
Disp

Medical

Daily prescription medicine
Required medical devices (glucose meters, blood pressure cuffs)
Children's medication
First aid kit (Appendix I)

Spare glasses, contact lenses, solution, cases
Spare hearing aids and batteries

Equipment
Flashlights and batteries
Portable radio and spare batteries
NOAA weather alert radio and batteries
Hammer, nails, saw, wrench, pliers, screwdriver, shovel
Plastic sheeting, tarps
Duct tape
Rugged "work" clothes to include gloves and boots
Plastic helmets, eye and ear protection
Dust masks
Sleeping bags
Fire Extinguisher

Paperwork
Small denomination bills and coins (cash)
Information Packet (Appendix D)
Local maps

B. Food

2 week home supply
Foods that require minimal preparation or clean up:

Pop Tarts
Granola Bars
Fruit juice
Canned goods
> Vegetables, fruit, sauces,
> Soups, ravioli, spaghetti
> Ham, tuna, salmon, chicken

Peanut butter
Jelly
Crackers
Comfort foods – candy, coffee, tea

Bug Out Bag food

Energy bars
Jerky
Peanuts
Dried Fruit
Peanut butter
Gatorade powder
MREs

Long Term Storage Food

Wheat
Dried Corn
White Rice
Pasta
Instant Cocoa, Tea, and Coffee
Oil
Salt

C. Evacuation (72 Hour) Kit

These kits can be used at home or taken with you during an evacuation. As such, they should be easy to access on the way out of the home and should be sized so that they are not too difficult to carry to the vehicle.

Containers – Tote bins and duffle bags work well
Bug out Bag per person (Appendix G)

Change of clothing
Information packet (Appendix D)
Cash in small denominations
Water – Three gallons per person
Food – Three supply per person (Appendix B)
First Aid Kit (Appendix I)
Tents
Sleeping bags and pads
Outdoor cooking gear
Cell phone and charger

D. Information Packet

*Some people keep important documents in a safe
deposit box – this is fine as long as you realize that you
may not always have access to your bank. Others keep
them in a firebox or in a safe at home. How ever you
store your documents, you should have copies made
of them so that you can keep Information Packets in
several places – such as your retreat location, your Bug
out Bag and so on. This information can be stored on a
laptop computer, on a memory stick, and/or on CDs but
you should also include paper backup copies.*

Family Contact Plan (Appendix K)

Xeroxed copies of credit cards

Identification (originals or copies)
      Drivers License
      Professional ID
      Birth Certificate
      Proof of address

Bank Account Numbers, Stocks, IRAs

Copy of Lease

Copy of Will, Powers of Attorney

Inventory of Possessions

Important phone numbers
    Hospital(s) *
    Fire Department *
    Police Desk *
    Insurance company
    Relatives, Friends, and Neighbors
  *(actual number other than 911)

Copies of Prescription Medicines, eyewear, or other medical devices

E. Kids Survival Supplies

Your child should have these things on their person whenever they are in the outdoors.
Proper Clothing
Whistle
Bright clothing or material
Large trash bag
Light
Snack
Fluids
Space blanket
First aid items
Cord

When they demonstrate they can properly and safely use them, add:
Lighter/Matches/Tinder
Pocket knife

F. BOV Equipment

Spare tire (in good condition) *consider having two*
Jack and lug wrench (consider a high lift jack)
Battery powered air compressor
Bicycle air pump
2 Quarts oil
1 Gallon antifreeze mix
1 Quart automatic transmission fluid (if needed)
1 Bottle power steering fluid (if needed)
Basic tools – pliers, screwdrivers, hammer, wrenches
Rag
Stiff wire
Duct tape
Spare belts and hoses (save your old ones)
Hose clamps
Empty gas can
Extra fuses
Leather Gloves
Head lamp
Winch or come-along
Tow straps
Clevis pins and shackles
Rope
Bow saw
Axe
Bolt cutters
D-handled shovel
Piece of carpet
Tire chains
Chilton's or like manual in waterproof bag
Maps
GPS
CB radio
Spot light

Maglite
Spare clothing
Water
Food
Sleeping bags or blankets
First aid kit
Binoculars

G. Bug Out Bag

*Every member of the family who can walk should have
their own. Items will be tailored according to physical
ability, age, climate, bug out plan, and so on. These are
just suggested items and areas to consider.*

Back Pack
Clothing bag (separate from BOB but attached)
      Long pants
      Long sleeved shirt
      T-shirt
      Under wear, socks
      Bandana
      Sturdy footwear
Additional clothing
      Jacket/coat
      Hat
      Rain gear
      Gloves
      Sweater

Canteen and water purification means (tablets, filter)
High energy food – Energy bars, jerky, peanut butter,
crackers, nuts
First Aid Kit – Ace bandages, tape, pain killers.
Shelter – tarp, poncho, or tent.
Sleeping bag or blanket

Maps, compass, GPS
Lighters, matches in waterproof container, tinder
Knife
Cordage
Repair gear
>   Duct tape
>   Wire
>   Sewing kit

Feminine Hygiene products
Copies of important papers and records
>   Marriage and birth certificates,
>   Inventories of household goods
>   Addresses and phone numbers of contacts and
>   family
>   Proof of address

Cash in smaller denominations
Spare glasses
Empty contact lens case and solution
Prescription or daily medications
Written prescriptions
Firearms and ammunition
Bible

Winter Gear
>   Long underwear
>   Sleeping bag
>   Sleeping pad
>   Backpacker stove and fuel bottle
>   Winter coat

Child's BOB

*These items should help keep a young child alive for a
period of time if they get separated from the main group.*

Small day pack

Poncho
Canteen
Food
Flashlight

As they get larger and or more mature/skilled you may add:
Sleeping bag
Knife
Firestarters
First aid items

Keep adding things as the child grows until they have their own "complete" BoB.

H. References

These are books I have acquired and read over the years and consider valuable references:

Nuclear War Survival Skills – Cresson Kearny
Surviving Doomsday – Bruce Clayton
Where there is no doctor – David Werner
Barefoot doctors manual – Running Press
Where there is no dentist – Murray Dickson
Back to Basics – Readers Digest
The truth about self protection – Massad Ayoob
Gun-Proof Your Children! – Massad Ayoob
To Ride, Shoot straight, and speak the truth – Jeff Cooper
Secure Home – Joel Skousen

I. Basic First Aid Kit

Latex gloves (or non-allergenic if you are allergic to latex)
Gauze dressings - 4x4 and 2x2
Triangular bandage
Ace Bandage
Adhesive tape
Scissors
Tweezers
Soap
Iodine and alcohol wipes
Antibiotic ointment
Burn ointment
Adhesive bandages (Band-Aids)
Eye wash solution
Thermometer
Prescription medications
Prescribed medical supplies (glucose meter, blood pressure cuff)
Tube of petroleum jelly or other lubricant
Aspirin and nonaspirin pain reliever/fever reducer
Anti-diarrhea medication
Antacid
Laxative

J. Family Contact Plan

_____ Mom's Cell
_____ Mom's Work
_____ Dad's Cell
_____ Dad's Work
_____ Son's Cell
_____ Daughter's Cell
_____ School Office
_____ Home
_____ Aunt Millie
_____ Grandpa Joe

1. Primary Plan is for Mom to pick children up (probably at school) and all meet at home.

2. Alternate Plans:
    A. In the event children must evacuate and flee from school, walk home via this route:
    (1). Head towards the football field
    (2). Go Left/West around the end zone and into the woods
    (3). Cut through the woods to Ash Street
    (4). Follow Ash street home

    B. Mom's pick up point is corner of 8th Street and Willow Ave in Walsh Drug Store

    C. Dad's pick up point is Fire Station on Johnston Road

3. Emergency Plan: Family will meet at church

4. Contingency Plan: Family will meet at Nelsons house:

    3422 S. Liberty Street
    Wasalooka, KS
    Phone: 822-555-1365

CPSIA information can be obtained
at www.ICGtesting.com
Printed in the USA
BVHW042050010820
585272BV00010B/162